Wei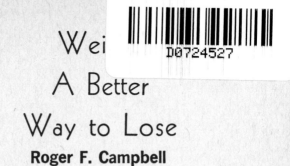 A Better Way to Lose

Roger F. Campbell

This book is designed for the reader's personal use and profit. It is also intended for group study. A leader's guide is available from your local Christian bookstore or from the publisher at $1.25.

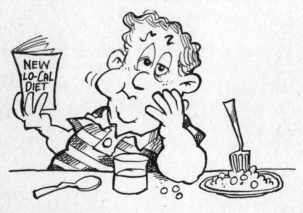

VICTOR BOOKS

a division of SP Publications, Inc., Wheaton, Illinois
Offices also in Fullerton, California • Whitby, Ontario, Canada • London, England

Fifth printing, 1978

Unless otherwise noted, Scripture quotations in this book are from *The New Scofield Reference* Bible, © 1967 by the Delegates of the Oxford University Press, Inc. Also used is *The Amplified Bible* (AMP) © by Zondervan Publishing House, Grand Rapids, Michigan.

Library of Congress Catalog Card Number: 76-14647
ISBN: 0-88207-735-X

VICTOR BOOKS
A division of SP Publications, Inc.
P.O. Box 1825 • Wheaton, Illinois 60187

Contents

Preface   **5**

1   Who Cares If I'm Fat?   **9**

2   Which Diet Works?   **19**

3   When You're Down You're Up!   **31**

4   The Devil Made Me Do It   **41**

5   Fat Faith   **51**

6   The Fruit That Makes You Thin   **61**

7   A Little Profit   **71**

8   Take the Plunge   **81**

9   Body Work   **93**

10   For Married Losers   **105**

11   Share Your Slimming Successes   **117**

12   Keep It Off by Keeping It Up   **123**

to
Pauline
who after 25 years of marriage
is still trim and beautiful

Preface

I believe the Bible contains the principles to solve every problem in life. Millions agree with me. In that Book they have found counsel and the power to set them free from sin and guilt. A host of harmful habits has fallen before its message. Shaky lives have found a firm foundation on which to plant their feet.

I had been in the ministry nearly 20 years, however, before I realized a sizable segment of my congregation was struggling with a serious problem that seemed unrelated to Bible truth. Alcoholics could be made sober. Drug addicts could be delivered. Prostitutes made pure. But the overweight appeared to be omitted from divine assistance. The more I thought about that the more sure I was that it could not be true.

As I studied the Scriptures that I felt might be related to the emotional and physical needs of the overweight person, I became convinced that the Christian life-style set forth in the Bible would, over a period of time, solve the dieter's dilemma. We therefore offered a weight-loss class in church; this book is a result of the success of that class.

If you want to lose 20 pounds in the next 10 days, our plan is not for you. Close the book. On the other hand, if you are fed up with the fat fads that have kept you losing one week and gaining the next, you may be ready for a permanent solution to your problem. It is my prayer that you will find it within the pages of this book.

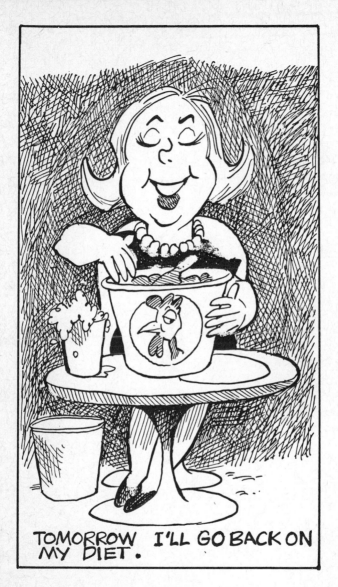

You are
the foot soldier
in the weight war.

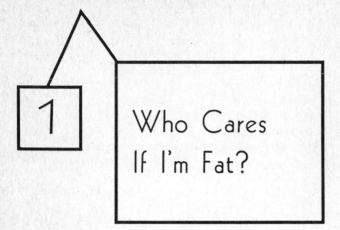

1 Who Cares If I'm Fat?

You say you want to lose weight? Welcome to the club. This is one battle you won't have to fight alone. The American Medical Association accepts as a reasonable estimate that three out of every five men and women in the United States are at least 10 percent above their desirable weight. Probably one out of three of these people is at least 20 percent above. It is no wonder, then, that about 100 million people in this weight-conscious country are on some kind of diet, fighting the battle of the bulge.

The passion to scale down has not gone unnoticed Fortunes are being made in the fat field. Sellers of diet foods are reaping a bonanza—$700 million last year. The gross profit margin on diet foods in supermarkets has been reported as 23 percent, one of the highest in the store. If you are "thinking thin" you can expect to be pampered, wooed, warned, and analyzed. And all for a profit! Reducing farms, exercise clubs, and diet doctors

9

represent only the tip of the iceberg in the multi-million dollar weight-control business.

On the other side of the profit-motive coin, some companies are offering incentives to employees who lose weight.

Jim Miller, president of Intermatic, Inc., a Spring Grove, Illinois electronics firm, believes that people of normal weight have more drive and more energy than people who are overweight. So, he's offering all his overweight employees $3 a pound for each pound of flab they shed during the year.

Lowe's Inc., of Cassopolis, Michigan—with $4 million annually in cat product sales—offers cash bonuses to executives who lose weight. President Edward Lowe started the ICATLYC, or "I Can't Afford To Lose You Club." Each member is given his optimum weight by the company doctor, and as many weeks as he has pounds to lose. If he makes the deadline, he is paid one-and-a-half percent of his annual salary, with the bonus renewed as long as he stays in trim. A $20,000-a-year man stands to gain $300 annually.

In six weeks 10 staffers lost a total of 80 pounds. Lowe figures such losses are gains, since for every executive who dies too soon, the company must spend twice his annual salary to train a replacement. Additional savings are expected from slimmer expense accounts.

Some care for cash.

Others care for you.

The Dangers of Obesity

If you are too heavy, it is likely those nearest you are concerned. They may not talk about it, for fear of offending you, but they care. The dangers of obesity are so well publicized that nearly everyone is aware of them. And they are for real!

Dr. Harry K. Panjwani, a consulting psychiatrist in Glen Rock, New Jersey, wrote of some of the emotional and physical pitfalls of that condition:

> The obese person usually feels unloved, unattractive, and unworthy. Deep within he may be wallowing in self-pity, jealousy, hostility, loneliness, and anger. He probably lives daily with depression, unhappiness, and frustration.
>
> In addition to the emotional burdens borne by those who are overweight, there are serious health risks: heart disease, high blood pressure, diabetes, strokes, and complications during pregnancy and childbirth." [1]

The Metropolitan Life Insurance Company put it this way: "For every inch your waist measurement exceeds your chest measurement, *subtract two years of your life.*"

A missionary who was overweight received a letter from one of her superiors that quickly changed her life-style and appearance. The letter simply expressed regret that the maxi-missionary would have such a short time to serve the Lord since her life would be shortened by her excess weight.

Dr. Ralph L. Byron, chairman of surgery at City of Hope Medical Center, Duarte, California said:

> Insurance statistics clearly tell the story: A person's life is shortened by one percent for each pound he is overweight. To illustrate, if a person of age 40 is 40 pounds overweight, his normal additional life expectancy of 40 years is cut off by 16 years.

The list of diseases which are influenced by being

---

[1] Dr. Harry K. Panjwani, "The Private Agony of the Obese," *Power For Living,* April 20, 1975.

overweight is long. Gallbladder disease, diabetes, and even cancer have a greater frequency among overweight individuals.

The strain on the heart, blood vessels, and lungs is even more closely related. Every pound of fat increases the miles of capillaries through which the heart must pump blood. The overweight person also has an increased tendency to arteriosclerosis.[2]

Those are dangers you can do without.

The Divine Dimension of Dieting

If you have been taking your weight lightly, it's time to face the facts.

There is someone who cares. His name is Jesus.

You knew that He was interested in your soul. But your size? It never entered your mind. Yet it should have, for the Bible teaches that God is concerned about our needs.

Jesus met the much-married woman at the well of Samaria and communicated with her about her thirst of body *and* soul (John 4:1-42).

Mary, listening at Jesus' feet, demonstrated a spiritual hunger. The Saviour commended her by saying she had chosen that good part, which would not be taken away from her (Luke 10:38-42). Spiritual gains are eternal.

The widow of Nain carried emotional and physical burdens. She was grieving because of the death of her son, and was without support through this loss. Jesus raised her son and dried her tears (7:11-18).

At the wedding in Cana, the people were out of wine. The problem was purely physical, yet it

---

[2] Dr. Ralph L. Byron, "Ask the Doctor," *Power For Living*, December 9, 1973.

brought forth the first recorded miracle of our Lord (John 2:1-12).

The point is that God is interested in you. He loves you, all of you: body, soul, and spirit. (See 1 Thes. 5:23.) He is not like the hypocrite who claims to love a man's soul but can't stand the rest of him. It is true that your spiritual needs have priority. You are to seek first the kingdom of God and His righteousness (Matt. 6:33), but stopping there embraces only half the truth.

Consider creation.

Everything in the universe, except the human frame, was simply spoken into existence. "And God said, 'Let the earth bring forth the living creature after its kind, cattle, and creeping things, and beast of the earth after its kind,' and it was so" (Gen. 1:24).

Not so the body of man. "And God said, 'Let us make man in our image, after our likeness; and let them have dominion over the fish of the sea, and over the fowl of the air, and over all the earth, and over every creeping thing that creepeth upon the earth'" (1:26). "And the Lord God formed man of the dust of the ground, and breathed into his nostrils the breath of life; and man became a living soul" (2:7).

The Psalmist David praised God for his body. He wrote: "I will praise Thee; for I am fearfully and wonderfully made" (Ps. 139:14).

When Christ came to this planet, the human body became His vehicle of redemption. He was "made in the likeness of men" (Phil. 2:7). He referred to His body as His temple. He said the resurrection of His body would be the proof of His deity (John 2:18-22).

The coming resurrection reveals divine regard for our bodies. Christ was resurrected bodily from the grave, just as we shall be at His coming. When that day arrives our bodies will be perfect without the aid of diets or doctors.

Till then, count calories.

Most encouraging to the Christian should be the fact that his/her body is the temple of God. The Bible teaches that the Holy Spirit actually lives within every believer. "What? Know ye not that your body is the temple of the Holy Ghost which is in you, which ye have of God, and ye are not your own? For ye are bought with a price; therefore, glorify God in your body and in your spirit, which are God's" (1 Cor. 6:19-20).

Now you have a divine dimension of dieting. Since your body is the Lord's temple, it should be kept in the best possible condition at all times. Some Christians miss this truth. They seem to think it carnal to care about personal appearance. To them, sloppiness and spirituality are somehow related. Weight control is something relegated to "the flesh." They leave the impression that their goals are higher.

These same people will work long and give sacrificially to make the local church building attractive. After all, it is the Lord's house, His temple. Yet, you search the New Testament in vain for that title given to a meeting place for the church. Your body is His temple. "Know ye not that ye are the temple of God, and that the Spirit of God dwelleth in you? If any man defile the temple of God, him will God destroy; for the temple of God is holy, which temple are ye" (1 Cor. 3:16-17).

The most fundamental reason for not conquering

your weight problem may be a mistaken separation of the physical and spiritual. To you, dedication has to do with: singing in the choir, going to church services, praying, reading the Bible, and witnessing to your neighbors. You have thought little about the importance of your body in carrying out these responsibilities. If your health fails, however, your opportunity for sacred service will be severely limited. You must remember that, to the Christian, everything is sacred. Commitment to Christ includes the dedication of your body. "I beseech you therefore, brethren, by the mercies of God, that ye present your *bodies* a living sacrifice, holy, acceptable unto God, which is your reasonable service" (Rom 12:1).

Since your body is the temple of the Holy Spirit, it is logical to conclude that His power is available for the purpose of keeping it in a condition that is pleasing to Him. It is His property. You can claim His power in your effort to take proper care of His temple.

Who cares if you're fat? Strange and exciting as it may seem, God cares.

The Human Dimension of Dieting

But there is another who must care if you are to achieve your goal in weight control. *You must care.* You are the foot soldier in this weight war. Without your effort the battle of the bulge will be lost.

So, the ball has just been tossed to you.

Do you *really* want to lose weight?

Is your appearance important to you?

Do you believe your weight is affecting your health?

Do you care about length of life?

Are you insecure because of your weight?

Do you envy people who always seem to look just right?

Are you now spending money to take off pounds?

Could your weight be affecting your Christian testimony?

Have you been guilty of neglecting God's temple?

If you find yourself giving an affirmative answer to most of these questions you may be ready for the most important question of all: Are you willing to change your life-style? If not, the biblical formula I am about to share with you will be little more than a reading exercise.

Five years from today you will probably be starting another grapefruit diet, or some other fruity fad. You will have bounced your way through a score of yo-yo experiences on the bathroom scales without getting one ounce closer to the answer you have been seeking. And, unless you have become an insurance statistic, you will be looking for some sure-fire way to become slim and trim.

On the other hand, you may finally be tired of the gimmicks and false promises of a thousand diets. You want the real thing, even if it involves a revolution in your way of life. If so, you are ready to lose weight.

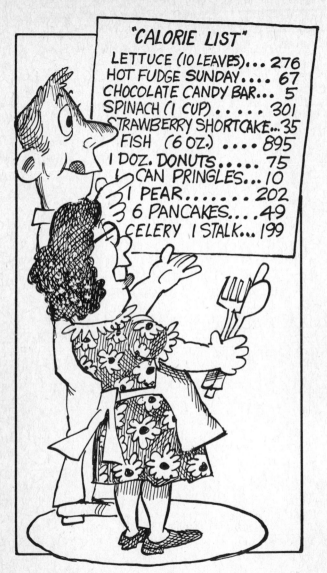

"CALORIE LIST"

LETTUCE (10 LEAVES)... 276
HOT FUDGE SUNDAY.... 67
CHOCOLATE CANDY BAR... 5
SPINACH (1 CUP) 301
STRAWBERRY SHORTCAKE...35
FISH (6 OZ.) 895
1 DOZ. DONUTS..... 75
1 CAN PRINGLES...10
1 PEAR........ 202
6 PANCAKES....49
CELERY 1 STALK...199

The average American
eats 100 pounds
of sugar per year . . .
taking in
174,600 calories

2 Which Diet Works?

Some scoff at the thought of ever living on a diet. Yet everyone does. A diet simply sets the limits on the type and quantity of food on which you live. Those limits may be very broad, or confined for a special purpose.

Diet Information in the Bible

Our first parents received a prescribed diet from their Creator. They were told that they could eat of every tree in the Garden of Eden, except one. Giving that one restriction, the Lord said, "But of the tree of the knowledge of good and evil, thou shalt not eat of it, for in the day that thou eatest thereof thou shalt surely die" (Gen. 2:17). Obedience, not obesity, was the issue when Adam and Eve disobeyed the Lord. Yet, food was a factor in that first temptation, and we should not forget it.

For their journey from Egypt to the promised land, the Children of Israel were given a diet of manna and meat. Both were miraculously supplied.

19

That miracle is described in Exodus 16:13-15: "And it came to pass that at evening the quails came up and covered the camp; and in the morning the dew lay round about the host. And when the dew that lay was gone up, behold, upon the face of the wilderness there lay a small round thing, as small as the hoar frost on the ground. And when the children of Israel saw it, they said one to another, 'It is manna': for they knew not what it was. And Moses said unto them, 'This is the bread which the Lord hath given you to eat.'"

Interestingly, as far as we know, this is the only time in history that men have shared the diet of angels (Ps. 78:25). While the immediate purpose of this heavenly diet was the survival of the Jews, Jesus revealed the deeper lesson contained in the miracle. He explained: "Your fathers did eat manna in the wilderness, and are dead. This is the bread that cometh down from heaven, that a man may eat of it, and not die. I am the living bread that came down from heaven; if any man eat of this bread, he shall live forever" (John 6:49-51).

Dietary laws were an important part of the instruction given to Moses for the people to observe in their new land. Especially concerning the eating of meats. They were allowed to eat any animal that parted the hoof and chewed the cud. Other animals were to be considered unclean. Great detail is also given as to the "clean" and "unclean" of fish and fowl. (See Deuteronomy 14:3-21.) These laws were to set the nation of Israel apart from the other nations.

Christians are not bound by these laws today. Paul declared, "Let no man, therefore, judge you in food, or in drink, or in respect of a feast day, or of the new moon, or of a sabbath day, which are a shadow of things to come; but the body is of Christ" (Col. 2:16-17). Nevertheless, they demonstrate the biblical principle of *special diets for certain worthwhile purposes.*

There are more examples worth noting.

As a Nazarite, Samson drank neither wine nor strong drink and abstained from eating any unclean thing (Jud. 13:4).

Daniel and his friends chose vegetarian fare instead of the meat that had been offered to Nebuchadnezzar's idols. At the end of ten days they were "fairer and fatter in flesh" than those who ordered from the king's menu (Dan. 1:15). While at this time "fat flesh" is anything but our goal, the principle stands.

John the Baptist lived on locusts and wild honey. That was an unusual diet, but John was an unusual man.

The Overweight Christian's Challenge

Paul said that he was willing to adjust his diet in any way necessary to keep from offending his brother. "Wherefore if food make my brother to offend, I will eat no meat while the world standeth, lest I make my brother to offend" (1 Cor. 8:13).

Are you willing to make that kind of commitment?

Bill Pauley was! At one time, Mr. Pauley, a minister, weighed 384 pounds and had a 58-inch waist. He said that buying a car was like buying a suit— he had to be fitted. When he wanted to weigh himself, he went to the butcher shop to use the scale. He recalled,

I will always remember the time I boarded the airplane and sat in one of those tight seats. I could hardly get into it. When the stewardess asked if my seatbelt was fastened, I told her I could not get it around me in the first place; and in the second place, if there were a crash, she would not have to worry—I would be stuck to the seat permanently!" [1]

For the most part, he had been able to laugh off his heavyweight appearance. He seems to have followed the if-you-have-a-lemon-make-lemonade policy, and had even developed a fine string of jokes about his weight to use as openers in his meetings. Then one day he found himself in a situation that wasn't funny.

While he was the speaker in youth meetings in central Illinois, he heard about a statement made by one of the teenage girls there. It was a shocker! She had said: "If Mr. Pauley can eat, then I can smoke."

Pauley's reaction? "For years I had criticized smoking and drinking and had preached the Word of God without applying the matter of temperance to myself. It was not until I heard what this girl had said that I became convicted of overeating."

William Pauley claimed the power of God and went on a diet. He lost 179 pounds and his waist went from 58 inches to 36 inches. He ended his weight problem.

Diets, Diets, Diets

Diets abound! They are offered everywhere. Magazines, newspapers, paperbacks, and hardcovers all

---

[1] William Pauley, "Mr. Before and After," *Power Life,* April 23, 1967.

get into the act. Such variety! Such confusion! Shall you choose:

The high protein diet or the high fat diet?

The high carbohydrate diet or the low carbohydrate diet?

The drinking man's diet or the thinking man's diet?

The grape diet or the grapefruit diet?

The one-meal-a-day diet or the nibbler's diet?

The calories-don't-count diet or the calorie counter's diet?

The one-food diet or the eat-whatever-you please diet?

And then there are the wild ones. One lady revealed she had eaten nothing but eggs on the first day of her diet. The next day she would eat only bananas. The third day, nothing but wieners. Frankly, I thought she was joking, but she was serious, as I think her condition would have been had she stayed long on that diet.

Weight loss is important, but it is not the only factor in choosing a diet. Your body must be nourished properly or you may also lose your health.

Most weight-loss diets seem to fall into one of three categories.

Into the fad diet group fall all the one-food and crash diets. Unless you have only a few pounds to lose I believe it is best to avoid these. It is not likely that you would be content to live for any long period of time on grapefruit, grapes, or rice. The monotony would be unbearable, not to mention the lack of balance for your body's needs. The will of God for man in the beginning seems to have been variety in his eating. "And the Lord God took man, and put him into the garden of Eden to till it and to keep it. And the Lord God commanded the man, saying, 'Of every tree of the garden thou mayest freely eat; but of the tree of the knowledge of good and evil, thou shalt not eat of it; for in the day that thou eatest thereof thou shalt surely die'" (Gen. 2:15-17).

The second diet division contains the low carbohydrate diets. These may be known by a number of different titles, such as: High Protein Diet, High Fat Diet, Meat and Cottage Cheese Diet. The discerning dieter, however, will notice that regardless of the title the result is the same. That being the reduction of his intake of carbohydrates.

Sugar is a carbohydrate, and when you consider the American appetite for sugar, it is understandable that most of us need to cut down in this area. Sugar contains four calories per gram, and we consume mountains of it. The average American eats 100 pounds of sugar per year. This means he takes in 174,600 calories which, if not burned up, add 50 pounds of extra weight.

Most carbohydrates are delicious, and some are necessary. It is easy to understand Solomon's counsel to his son: "My son, eat thou honey, because it is good, and the honeycomb, which is sweet to thy taste" (Prov. 24:13). We should also give attention to this advice: "It is not good to eat much honey" (25:27).

Because I have hypoglycemia (low blood sugar), I have to live on a low carbohydrate diet. I had no idea of the tremendous amount of carbohydrates in my way of life until I was forced to cut them.

My practice had been to start each morning with coffee, cereal, and toast. The coffee and cereal were sugared to my taste and the toast liberally spread with jelly. In mid-morning I had coffee and a glazed donut. Lunch was capped with cookies or cake, when possible. My sweet tooth demanded attention at some time during the afternoon, and dinner was best when rounded out with a piece of my favorite pie. Most any kind of pie is my favorite. Evening snack time usually meant ice cream or some similar calorie carrier. Though weight had not become a real problem (my wife said you could only tell by hugging), my waist had expanded by four inches, and I believe the future might have found me a well-rounded personality, had not my eating habits changed.

The diagnosis of low blood sugar demanded an end to my sugar spree. I was told to remove all high carbohydrate foods from my diet, and I have done so. I do not eat pie, cake, cookies, or other such goodies. I abstain from all soft drinks that contain sugar, and I use no sweetener in my coffee. I eat few potatoes.

By now someone is feeling sorry for me. Don't! There are hundreds of mouth-watering morsels available to me. I can eat steaks, chops, seafoods, poultry, vegetables, most dairy products, and many fruits. All in sufficient quantity. It is a way of life that allows a great variety of healthful and enjoyable food. The following is a sample diet on an average day:

Breakfast	Eggs with ham, bacon, or sausage
	Toast—one slice with peanut butter
	Decaffeinated coffee—without sugar
	Fruit—unsweetened
Midmorning	Low fat milk

Lunch	Meat
	Salad
	Cottage cheese
	One slice of bread with butter
	Decaffeinated coffee—without sugar
Midafternoon	Low fat milk
Dinner	Meat—generous portion
	Vegetable
	Salad
	Cottage cheese and unsweetened fruit
	One slice of bread with peanut butter
	Decaffeinated coffee without sugar
Evening snack	Cold cuts
	Salad or cottage cheese with fruit

Though I was not trying to lose weight, this diet, along with my active schedule, dropped 30 pounds off my weight in one year. In fact, I have had to increase my quantity of food just to maintain my weight. The weight loss was due to the reduced intake of carbohydrates. Recently my doctor again advised me, "Keep shoveling that food in!"

Wouldn't you like to have that kind of medical advice? A low carbohydrate diet might make it possible.

Most other plans for losing weight fall into the calorie-counting company. This method of slimming down offers the most variety and demands the most discipline. Coupled with a proper exercise plan, it is a good way to lose weight.

Contrary to the contention of some recent magazine articles and books, calories do count. Dr. Jean Mayer, professor of nutrition at Harvard says: "Instead of backing into dieting by following a fad, why not begin where you will end up anyway—counting calories." [2]

Dr. Mayer has a point. Even the low carbohydrate and high protein diets are but other approaches to cutting calories. By reducing foods that pile up calories fast, and substituting others, the result is a lower calorie intake. If the exercise balance is right, this should then bring the desired weight loss.

Helps for the calorie counter are easily available. Books listing nearly all foods and giving calorie content are to be found in most bookstores, pharmacies, and many food stores. They are worth the investment.

The American Medical Association says a person leading a moderately active life needs 15 calories per pound each day. You should find out the approximate number of calories you need to hold your present weight. That may take some experimenting over a period of a few weeks. Then you can drop below that to lose. Hopefully.

It is generally true that a cut of 500 calories a day will bring about a weight loss of a pound a week. If you drop 1,000 calories a day, you should lose two pounds a week. You should not go below 1,200 calories a day unless you have been told to do so by your doctor. If you get too lo-cal, there is danger of depriving your body of necessary vitamins and minerals.

---

[2] Dr. Jean Mayer, "Calories Still Count," *Family Health*, October 1974, p. 42.

"A nice lot of information," you say, "but, back to the question: Which diet works?"

Any diet will work that reduces your calorie intake below what you burn in daily activity. Sound simple? It is. But there is one complicating factor: You. All diets fail without *you.* And here you are discouraged! You have tried before and failed. You have consulted your doctor, as you should, and are still overweight. You have had the best of intentions in the past, to no avail.

Take heart. It is to you that this unique study is directed. Help has arrived. Past failure is not a factor. Success in slimming is within your reach. This time is different. The difference is God. He offers the secret of control. His Word unfolds a *life-style* that will enable you to arrive at your goal, even in this difficult area of life.

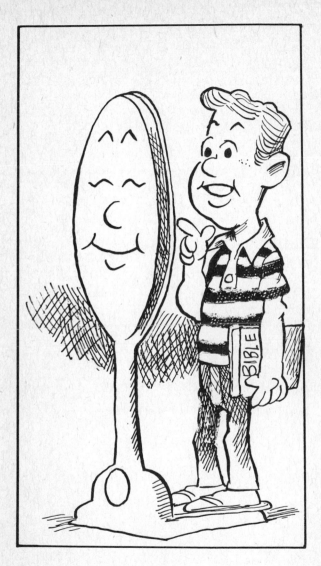

A heavy heart
weighs more
than you can afford.

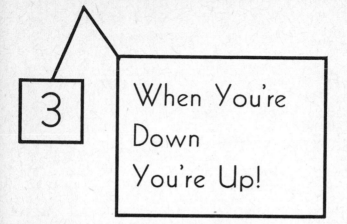

When You're Down You're Up!

3

Make no mistake—losing weight is a major undertaking. It involves the consuming of flesh and fiber of your body. And every ounce goes kicking and screaming. It is not surprising, then, that attitude must be right or failure is sure.

In this venture especially, "A merry heart doeth good like a medicine: but a broken spirit drieth the bones" (Prov. 17:22).

It is a well-known fact that depression adds to the weight problem. That state of mind saps strength and makes self-discipline difficult. In addition, the discouraged person often snacks to get his mind off his problems. Finally, gloom slows him down in all his actions and he does not burn up energy as he ought.

A Word from the Doctors

Dr. Harry K. Panjwani illustrated depression's defeating cycle with the case history of one of his patients:

31

When Maria (not her real name) came for her first appointment, she was the typical, overweight, unhappy woman. She was filled with anxieties and extremely depressed.

I found her to be a sensitive, passive, generous, and kind person. She had always had difficulty in asserting herself, and because of this others had often taken advantage of her. To console herself she usually indulged in food, tears, and self-pity.[1]

There must be millions of Marias.

Psychiatrist O. Quentin Hyder also accuses depression as one of the culprits causing obesity.

There are of course a few medical causes of obesity such as hormone imbalance and certain metabolic disorders. These need to be fully investigated and treated by a physician. The vast majority of causes, however, are neurotic.

Emotional deprivation often leads directly to the practice of eating as a substitute for the needed love and affection. It often starts in the unwanted child or one not given enough mother love. Adolescent girls who are afraid of relationships with the opposite sex allow themselves to get fat as a protection from being dated. They support their self-esteem by believing that all they need to do is lose weight and they will be very attractive. In fact, however, they are afraid to lose weight because of the deeply suppressed fear that if they did they might find out that after all, they were not so attractive as they thought.

Frustration, poor self-image, hostility, resentment, and depression are all neurotic problems related to a tendency to overeat. To many miserable people the

---

[1] Panjwani, "The Private Agony of the Obese."

simple fact of eating is the only pleasure they have in life.

In excess this is the sin of gluttony.[2]

Causes of Depression

Since being down keeps your weight up, it is essential to discover the causes of your depression and either conquer or avoid them. The Bible helps us understand some of the dynamics of depression.

You may be depressed because of fear.

Elijah was one of the most powerful prophets. He was a man of great courage. He was mighty in prayer. On one occasion he called down fire from heaven (1 Kings 18:36-38), and on another he raised the dead (17:22). His rank was such that he appeared with Moses on the mount of transfiguration (Matt. 17:3). Many expect him to return to earth in the future as one of the two witnesses mentioned in the Book of the Revelation (11:3). Still, fear drove him to despair. Threatened by Jezebel he moaned, "It is enough! Now O Lord, take away my life; for I am not better than my fathers" (1 Kings 19:4).

Like Elijah, you may be defeated by your fears. You wonder if life is worth living. You fear the future. You fear for your family. You fear that you may lose your financial security. You have fears about your health. You fear death.

No wonder you have not been able to control your weight. Your self-discipline is decimated by fear. Everything else is low priority compared to the catastrophes you expect to strike.

[2] From *The Christian's Handbook of Psychiatry* by O. Quentin Hyder, M.D. Copyright © 1971 by Fleming H. Revell Company. Used by permission.

What can you do? You can evaluate your fears. Of the things that you fear, how many are really likely to happen to you today? If you can feel safe for the remainder of the day, that is enough for now. Jesus said, "Be, therefore, not anxious about tomorrow; for tomorrow will be anxious for the things of itself. Sufficient unto the day is its own evil" (Matt. 6:34).

Which of your fears tormented you yesterday? Last week? Last year? Have you been down this road before? How many times have you been troubled by the same thought pattern that paralyzes you today, only to find that your expected tragedy never occurred? Can you believe that God will continue to protect you? Long ago, John Newton concluded:

> Thru many dangers, toils and snares
> I have already come;
> 'Tis grace hath brought me safe thus far,
> And grace will lead me home.

The grace of God is not diminished. It is as sufficient for you now as it was for Newton in his day.

What do you fear that is so serious it is not covered by one of the promises of God? Fear is not new. It is as old as sin. It was not long after the fall that Adam confessed that he was afraid: "And he said, I heard Thy voice in the garden, and I was afraid, because I was naked; and I hid myself" (Gen. 3:10). Your fears have not taken God by surprise.

My work constantly brings me into contact with people in the crisis hours of their lives. I am often there when the worst seems probable. I have learned that the promises given in the Bible are the best antidote for fear. Exposure to the Word of God builds faith, and when faith comes, fear leaves. The prophet Isaiah said, "Thou wilt keep him in perfect peace, whose mind is stayed on Thee, because he trusteth in Thee" (26:3).

Prayer also conquers fear. George Mueller, faced with the feeding of hundreds of orphans, must have been tempted to fear for provision of food many times. Yet prayer sustained him and chased his fears away. He explained: "I spend hours in prayer every day. But I live in the spirit of prayer. I pray as I walk and when I lie down. I pray when awake. The answers are always coming. Thousands of times have my prayers been answered. When I am persuaded that a thing is right, I go on praying until the answer comes." [3]

Give your fears to the Lord in prayer. That is what the psalmist did when he was troubled. And it worked. "I sought the Lord, and He heard me, and delivered me from all my fears" (Ps. 34:4). It will work for you.

You may be depressed because of unconfessed sin.

David had once been known for his merry heart. He was the singer of sweet songs. The composer of hymns of praise and thanksgiving. In his youth he was so gifted at driving away gloom that King Saul often summoned him to play and sing for him when he was depressed (1 Sam. 16:23). He had known the thrill of leading victorious armies. The adoration of women and children had lifted his

---

[3] Walter B. Knight, *Knight's Treasury of Illustrations*, (Grand Rapids, Mich.: William B. Eerdmans Publishing Co., 1963), p. 269.

heart when returning from battle as the conquering hero of Israel (18:6-7).

Yet, David also knew what it was to walk through the valley of despair. He was acquainted with depression. One day he lamented: "I sink in deep mire where there is no standing; I am come into deep waters, where the floods overflow me. I am weary of my crying. My throat is dried, mine eyes fail while I wait for my God" (Ps. 69:2-3).

What was it that had brought David down to the depths? What had stolen his song? We are not left to wonder. He had tried to cover his sin. Read his description of that awful time: "When I kept silence, my bones became old through my roaring all day long. For day and night Thy hand was heavy upon me; my moisture is turned into the drought of summer" (32:3-4).

His joy had disappeared. He felt tired and old. The man who had written: "My cup runneth over" (23:5), now seemed bankrupt of blessing. Many have sought peace without being willing to face their sins and confess them to the Lord. That approach to life's greatest issue can only result in more depression.

Thankfully, there is a pleasant ending to David's experience: "I acknowledged my sin unto Thee, and mine iniquity have I not hid. I said, 'I will confess my transgressions unto the Lord'; and Thou forgavest the iniquity of my sin" (32:5).

A wise move. And workable today: "If we confess our sins, He is faithful and just to forgive us our sins, and to cleanse us from all unrighteousness" (1 John 1:9).

Getting rid of that load could be your key to success in slimming.

You may be depressed because you have not accepted yourself.

You wish you were someone else. You envy the appearance and talents of others. You feel inferior. On your "down days," Proverbs 30:2 describes your self-image: "Surely I am more stupid than any man."

Low self-esteem is deceiving. Sometimes it parades as humility and expects commendation. Actually, it is rebellion against a wise Creator who formed and fashioned you according to His will.

I visited a man a number of times in an effort to win him to Christ. He had been quite successful, but now was rather withdrawn from social contacts. He always seemed to appreciate my visits and concern, yet he would not respond to my message.

Finally I discovered the reason. He was afraid by "receiving Christ" he would lose his individuality. He thought he would be "just another Christian." Part of the church group. Lumped together with the rest of the saved. One of the crowd headed for heaven.

Nothing could be farther from the truth.

It is true that God loves the world, but He loves men as individuals. He loves you. He has a plan for your life. There is a place for you in the Body of Christ that no one else can fill. Your gifts and talents are given so that you can carry out your individual role in the church. You are equipped exactly as God intended. Paul wrote to the Corinthian Christians: "For the body is not one member, but many. If the foot shall say, 'Because I am not the hand, I am not of the body,' is it, therefore not of the body? And if the ear shall say, 'Because

I am not the eye, I am not the body'; is it, therefore, not of the body? If the whole body were an eye, where were the hearing? If the whole were hearing, where were the smelling? But now hath God set the members, every one of them, in the body, as it hath pleased Him" (1 Cor. 12:14-18).

When my friend saw this, he was immediately ready to take Christ as his Lord and Saviour. It is a great truth. Accept it! You are important to God.

You may be depressed because you are hungry.

A strange statement to find in a book about losing weight. Yet, it is often true.

Some can go without food for long periods of time with little emotional effect. Others cannot. You may be one who drops into the doldrums when your body runs low on fuel. When that happens you raid the refrigerator and blow your diet.

You can't understand it. You've read the articles about the advantages of eating one meal a day. Your friends recommend it. What's wrong? Must be your poor will power! Perhaps not! Here comes that individuality again. Now you know why it is so difficult to come up with a diet that works for everyone. We are not all the same. Some burn calories fast, while others get better mileage.

If you are a fast burner and feel down when you abstain from food over a period of hours, I suggest that you eat when you are hungry. Not those carload-of-calories snacks, of course. You will have to avoid them. But there are plenty of nourishing foods that add few calories. Low-fat milk works well for me. Skimmed milk is loaded with protein and is not likely to add weight. Celery or carrot sticks are satisfying. Your calorie counter's book will allow you to find a number of healthful, en-

Sounds sound. But is there a Bible basis for Lovett's logic? There is.

The Devil's Purpose—Destruction

The first temptation involved food. Satan's strategy in his approach to Eve is preserved for us in Genesis 3:1: "Yea, hath God said, Ye shall not eat of every tree of the garden?" The fact was that our first parents were allowed to eat anything in the garden except the fruit of one tree. That provided them with immense variety. There should have been no problem in avoiding the forbidden fruit. Yet, Satan was able to turn Eve's attention away from all that God had given to focus on the one restriction.

Many diets die that death. One slice of devil's food cake (well-named) becomes more important than pounds or peace of mind. Truckloads of nourishing food could not compete with that one delicious desert. One bite and all is lost—except weight.

The real purpose of our enemy, of course, was the destruction of God's creation. That goal has not changed. A study of the devil and demonism reveals satanic design to injure or destroy our bodies.

Job was both healthy and wealthy before his encounter with Satan. As the result of Satan's attack upon him, he lost everything, including his health. The origin of Job's agony is revealed in one short verse: "So went Satan forth from the presence of the Lord, and smote Job with sore boils from the sole of his foot unto his crown" (Job 2:7).

In Job's case, yielding to temptation was not the cause of his misery. There was nothing he could have done to prevent his problems. The tragedy it-

joyable snack foods that will boost you over the hungry times.

Enduring depression to lose weight is not part of this program. Conquering, or avoiding it, is.

You may be depressed because you are overweight.

"Finally," you say, "I wondered how long you would beat around the bush. Every time I look in the mirror I'm depressed."

Exactly. And that sets up that awful cycle mentioned at the beginning of this chapter. Your weight makes you depressed. You eat because you are depressed, and that increases your weight, creating deeper depression.

Together we are going to break that cycle. You have been on the merry-go-round long enough. You will adopt a new life-style that will trim inches from your waist and drop pounds off your frame. But it will help greatly if you can discover the reason for your depression. If you have not identified with one of the causes presented here, visit a Christian bookstore and take advantage of the excellent material now available to help the depressed person. I especially recommend Tim LaHaye's *How to Win over Depression* (Zondervan Publishing House).

Some who suffer from severe chronic depression may need to seek professional counseling. If that is your case, do so. It will be worth it.

A heavy heart weighs more than you can afford.

Satan was able
to turn Eve's attention
away from all that
God had given to focus
on the one restriction.
Many diets die
that death.

4 The Devil Made Me Do It

"Can the devil make us fat?" That is the question posed by well-known author C. S. Lovett.

It's a question worth considering.

"Oh, come now," you say. "What interest does the devil have in my weight?"

A great deal, according to Lovett.

Satan works overtime to get us to overeat. He knows what extra pounds can do to the body and mind of a believer. While some people seemingly get away with being oversize, most do not. Extra fat makes many of us look ugly. What's worse, it drains our energy, loads up the heart making us more susceptible to disease—including cancer. While some are able to ride out the psychological problems this creates, most are defeated by them. That's when Satan whispers, "If the Lord can't give you victory in something like this, how can you expect victory in other areas?" [1]

---

[1] C. S. Lovett, *Personal Christianity*, February 1974.

self was his test. However, this is the exception rather than the rule, and the lesson is in the devil's delight in robbing a man of his health.

A number of accounts of bodily injury or illness caused by satanic power are recorded in the New Testament. Typical is the case encountered by Jesus and the disciples after they descended from the mountain of transfiguration. There they met a desperate father who begged them to help his son. Dr. Luke's description is worth noting: "And, behold, a man of the company cried out, saying, 'Master, I beseech Thee, look upon my son; for he is mine only child. And, lo, a spirit taketh him, and he suddenly crieth out; and it teareth him so that he foameth again and, bruising him, hardly departeth from him" (Luke 9:38-39).

It is clear that we face· a cruel enemy who is bent on our destruction and pleased with our misery. Jesus summarized Satan's purpose: "The thief cometh not but to steal, and to kill, and to destroy" (John 10:10).

He may kill with calories. Don't cooperate with him. If you still doubt that the devil is a weight-watcher, consider his other gains when you stuff yourself.

Your intemperance with food makes you disobedient to the Word of God: "Be not among wine-bibbers, among gluttonous eaters of flesh; for the drunkard and the glutton shall come to poverty" (Prov. 23:20-21).

Overeating is one of the more respectable sins in our society. Some Christians even boast of their great capacity for food, not imagining that drunkards and gluttons are relegated to the same company in the Scriptures.

Emotional hang-ups from being overweight can hinder Christian service. You may feel self-conscious about being before crowds because you are not happy with your appearance. You lack confidence, so you withdraw. You are no longer active in your church. The devil has you where he wants you.

To quote Lovett again:

It's one of God's laws that obedience brings blessing. But who feels like working for Christ with his vigor and vitality drained off by the extra weight? Fat Christians not only forfeit the *pep* and *zip* that go with a trim body, they are also denied the joy they could have serving Christ. It's not hard to see why Satan schemes to get Christians to eat more than they should. If he can make believers overweight and joyless, he can slow down the Christian program.[2]

In limiting your service and stifling the use of your talents and abilities you make it that much easier to gain more weight. It is another of the discouraging cycles of obesity. A cycle that you can conquer through Christ.

And then there is your money. You must know that Satan is interested in keeping your cash from fulfilling one of its highest purposes—investment in meeting the needs of a troubled world.

Obesity is expensive. Believe it or not, each calorie that contributed to your condition cost something. It is true that: "There is no such thing as a free lunch." You bought your bulges.

Not only that, you have probably spent plenty trying to get rid of your extra weight. Diet pills,

---

[2] C. S. Lovett, *Personal Christianity*, February 1974.

doctor's advice, exercise club memberships, uncounted magazines with diet information, may all have been a part of your struggle to be slim. All cost money.

Don't you think it's time to cut the fat out of your budget?

The Stewardship of Eating

One Christian lady recently became concerned with her stewardship in this part of her life. She decided she would eliminate the snacks and sweets that had kept her defeated, and for each of these she skipped, she would deposit the cost of that food in a fund to be given to the Lord's work. Imagine her double delight as she saw the fund growing and the fat going.

The issue of stewardship is an old one. The list of Christian taboos has always been beefed up with things considered a waste of money. And properly so. But what about all those rich goodies that seem to be a must at every gathering for fellowship? How much of that waste becomes waist? If we were to cash in our calories, I wonder how many it would take to support a missionary. The devil must smile at our double standards.

Another dimension to stewardship is that of sharing food with those who are hungry. That is a Christian responsibility. It even includes the feeding of our enemies: "Therefore, if thine enemy hunger, feed him" (Rom. 12:20).

There are many hungry in our world today. Dr. W. Stanley Mooneyham pointed this out.

> In recent months I have spent a lot of time among hungry and dying children on three continents. What I have seen causes me to raise up my voice

and weep until I have no more strength to weep.
In Bangladesh, I talked with a father of six. His
babies each eat one spoonful of rice a day. This
father told me that his wife was already dead, along
with half of his children. "My babies and I will soon
be dead also," he said.[3]

His heart heavy over the needs of the starving,
Dr. Jack Van Impe begged,

In the name of Jesus who loved little children, will
you please care, Christian? In Haiti, India, Brazil,
and Bangladesh, half of the children die before the
age of ten. Two hundred fifty million little children
are starving along with 550 million adults on a
world-wide scale. Should they feel like the psalmist
who said in chapter 142:4, "No man cared for my
soul," or can be assured that *you* care? [4]

The thought of millions of Christians really caring and sharing is exciting. What a great impact
the message of salvation would have if accom-
panied with the kind compassion Jesus demonstrated! You can be sure that Satan does not want
that to happen. He will be pleased to have us go
in our self-satisfied way, caring only for ourselves
and those nearest us.

But it does not have to be that way. You can
care.

Try this heavy thought: You can transfer those
unwanted pounds to some starving frame. You can
give them to someone who needs them. If you do
not know any hungry people, there are missionary
relief organizations within the mail reach of every

---

[3] Dr. W. Stanley Mooneyham, *The Jack Van Impe Crusade Newsletter,* September 1975.

[4] Dr. Jack Van Impe, *The Jack Van Impe Crusade Newsletter,* August 1975.

Christian in America who will be delighted to assist you in your pound-exchange project. You may be far more imaginative in developing this area of stewardship than I have been in making suggestions. I hope so.

The Devil Likes You Fat

It should be clear by now that you can expect satanic opposition in your effort to get in shape. Let's summarize the reasons:

1. The devil wants to ruin your health.
2. The devil want you to be disobedient to God's Word.
3. The devil wants to keep you from Christian service.
4. The devil wants to sidetrack Christian stewardship.

Since the devil wants to keep you fat, how can you ever hope to achieve your goal of losing weight? There can be but one answer. You must tap the resources available to you in Jesus Christ. Satan is too strong an enemy for you to face alone. In that kind of confrontation, you are sure to lose. And in this particular battle, when you lose, you gain.

Be encouraged, however, with the truth that you have a victorious Saviour. He has engaged the enemy and overcome him. Consider the temptation of Jesus. Interestingly, the first phase of that temptation had to do with food. "Then was Jesus led up by the Spirit into the wilderness to be tested by the devil. And when He had fasted forty days and forty nights, He was afterward hungry. And when the tempter came to Him, he said, 'If Thou be the Son of God, command that these stones be made bread'" (Matt. 4:1-3).

Unlike Eve, who was surrounded with plenty, Jesus had not eaten for 40 days, and there was no food in sight. In this setting, Satan's aim was the disqualifying of our Saviour so that man could not be redeemed. He failed, and the tempted can find in Jesus the One who understands their appetites, yet provides victory.

There in that barren place, tempted to change stones into bread, Jesus answered: "It is written, 'Man shall not live by bread alone, but by every word that proceedeth out of the mouth of God'" (Matt. 4:4).

No wonder the enemy was defeated! The living Word and the written Word were too much for him. That powerful combination is available to you, making it possible to be victorious in every area of life.

I know you have struggled long and hard with these temptations. You are war weary. You wonder if it is worth another battle. But this time, equipped by the Omnipotent, you are going to win.

And lose.

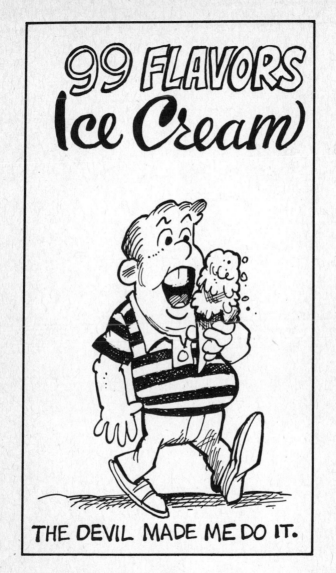

99 FLAVORS
Ice Cream

THE DEVIL MADE ME DO IT.

You have
too much to lose
by not losing
. . . your health,
your happiness,
and your future.

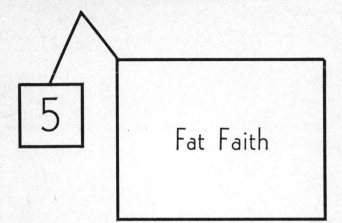

5

Fat Faith

A friend of mine who tips the scales at 295 insists that at the resurrection we'll discover the perfect weight to be 300 pounds.

Fat chance!

Still, there is a perfect weight for you. And that should be your goal. Picture yourself in that ideal form. You can be what you want to be. Jesus said, "If thou canst believe, all things are possible to him that believeth" (Mark 9:23).

Achieving an ideal weight seemed impossible to Charlie Shedd. He wrote:

Fifteen years and one hundred twenty pounds ago, I dropped to my knees and prayed: "Lord, I've tried for years to whip this problem of obesity. I've been on banana diets and eaten red meat. I've taken pills and bought reducing belts. I've read books, attended lectures, joined clubs, enrolled in courses. But I'm still fat. I weigh much too much. And I need help. In the Good Book you promise if anyone has enough faith he can say to a mountain, 'Go away,' and it will go. There's a mountain of flesh on me. I've been trying to move it ever since I was a boy. I've been laughed at. I've been ridiculed. I've rationalized. I've lied. I've had times when I cared and times when I didn't.

"I've decided to quit and promised I'd be good. Then we were invited out, and this woman makes the best biscuits. I've sworn off, and before I knew it, I found myself sitting at the fountain lapping a milk shake.

"Now I mean business. I accept You at Your word. Today I say to this mountain, 'Get moving.' I have faith that the two of us can move it together. This is the big surrender. I'm turning my body over to you once and for all. I can't manage it alone. From this day on, I'll eat what You tell me to eat and live how You want me to live. Amen." [1]

Shedd shed his flab with a life-style that is anchored in faith. So can you.

It would not be surprising to find that the good things in life come the faith route. You received salvation through faith: "For by grace are ye saved through faith" (Eph. 2:8).

Before that day of peace with God arrived you struggled and tried to find the answer to life, but to no avail. Neither religion nor ritual met your need. Finally faith made the difference: "Therefore being justified by faith, we have peace with God through our Lord Jesus Christ" (Rom. 5:1).

But faith is more than the key to eternal life. It is to be the daily experience of the child of God: "Now the just shall live by faith" (Heb. 10:38).

---

[1] *The Fat Is In Your Head* by Charlie Shedd. Copyright © 1972. Used by permission of Word Books, Publisher, Waco, Texas.

That verse caught fire in Martin Luther's heart and sparked the Reformation. Shaped the world. There must be power enough there to get you in shape.

The Bible defines faith as the "substance of things hoped for, the evidence of things not seen" (Heb. 11:1). Simply stated, that means being sure of the things you hope for and being settled in your conviction of their reality. In other words, it is being dead sure that God will grant your desire.

Dr. V. Raymond Edman, former president and late chancellor of Wheaton (Ill.) College, said this about faith: "Faith is dead to doubts, dumb to discouragements, blind to impossibilities, knows nothing but success. Faith lifts its hands up through the threatening clouds, lays hold of Him who has all power in heaven and on earth. Faith makes the uplook good, the outlook bright, the inlook favorable, and the future glorious." [2]

Now what do you want to weigh? Pray about it. Claim it. Expect it. Attain it.

Does this mean that faith will zap those extra pounds off overnight? Not quite. It does mean that you will tackle your problem with absolute confidence that you will win this time.

The Development of Faith

Great faith is built on the conviction that God can do anything. Most Christians believe that, but do not act on it. They accept omnipotence intellectually, but it makes little difference in their lives. Consequently, problems loom large, burdens become heavy, and the future is faced with fear.

---

[2] Knight, *Knight's Treasury of Illustrations*, p. 115.

Most of us need the challenge given to Jeremiah: "Behold, I am the Lord, the God of all flesh; is there anything too hard for me?" (Jer. 32:27) A. B. Simpson put his finger on the problem when he said, "Our God has boundless resources. The only limit it in us. Our asking, our thinking, our praying are too small. Our expectations are too limited." [3] J. Hudson Taylor also pointed to the problem. "Many Christians estimate difficulties in the light of their own resources, and thus atempt little and often fail in the little they attempt. All God's giants have been weak men who did great things for God because they reckoned on His power and presence with them." [4]

The New Testament abounds with miracles and promises that confirm the limitless power of God. The greatest of these is the incarnation of Jesus Christ. When the angel Gabriel appeared to Mary with the message that she would bear a son, and that He would be called the Son of the Highest, she couldn't understand it. She questioned: "How shall this be, seeing I know not a man?" (Luke 1:34) The angel assured Mary that with God, *nothing is impossible* (1:37). That exciting thought places everything within the reach of faith.

So you can attain your goal. Your past failures are not a factor. God is able, and His power is available. He will give you the ability to resist and to win.

The most tempting foods will lose their power to lure you from the path of success. Strawberry shortcake will surrender. Hot fudge sundaes will

---

[3] Knight, *Knight's Treasury of Illustrations*, p. 266.
[4] Knight, *Knight's Treasury of Illustrations*, p. 262.

melt away. Danish pastries will be foreign to your way of life. Discipline will be yours. Finally you will be free from that unwanted load that saps your strength and eats away at your emotional well-being.

Settle it. God is able to help you.

Faith is developed by exposure to the Bible. It cannot be pumped up; it cannot be faked. Its source is the Scriptures: "So then faith cometh by hearing, and hearing by the Word of God" (Rom. 10:17).

God's promises encourage faith. As you take time to study the Bible you will find guarantees of strength, peace, courage, salvation, power, victory, and answered prayer. You will read of the exploits of others who have conquered through faith. As you identify with these promises and personal triumphs, your faith will increase. Depression will depart. Expectation will emerge. You will know that you can become what you want to be.

Like most things, faith grows with exercise. David was able to face Goliath because he had already conquered wild beasts that attacked his father's sheep. By the time Moses lifted his rod and parted the Red Sea, he had witnessed the power of God in bringing the plagues on Egypt. The falling of the walls of Jericho came *after* Joshua had led his people through the river Jordan.

If you want to increase your faith you must start using the faith you now have. Do something that demands faith. Trust God for something that no one else can do for you. Flex your spiritual muscles. Expect God to honor His commitments. You'll be thrilled with the results. Spurgeon once said: "A little faith will bring your soul to heaven, but great faith will bring heaven to your soul." *Desire great faith more than you desire good food.*

Prove Your Faith

Dr. A. W. Tozer contrasted real faith with what he called "pseudo faith." He explained:

We can prove our faith by our committal to it and in no other way. Any belief that does not command the one who holds it is not a real belief; it is a pseudo belief only. And it might shock some of us profoundly if we were brought suddenly face to face with our beliefs and forced to test them in the fires of practical living.

Many of us Christians have become extremely skillful in arranging our lives so as to admit the truth of Christianity without being embarrassed by its implications. We arrange things so that we can get on well enough without divine aid, while at the same time ostensibly seeking it. We boast in the Lord but watch carefully that we never get caught depending on Him.

Pseudo faith always arranges a way out to serve in case God fails it. Real faith knows only one way and gladly allows itself to be stripped of any second way or makeshift substitutes. For true faith, it is either God or total collapse. And not since Adam first stood up on earth has God failed a single man or woman who trusted Him.[5]

So, get out on a limb with Jesus. Burn your bridges behind you. Tell your friends and family that you are going to get to the weight and appearance that you have wanted for so long. Let it

---

[5] Taken from *The Root of the Righteous* by A. W. Tozer and used by permission of Christian Publications, Inc., Harrisburg, Pa. 17101.

be known that you are trusting the Lord to give you the courage and discipline necessary to accomplish your goal.

Refuse to consider failure. Think only of success. Paul had something to say about filling the mind with positive things: "Finally, brethren, whatever things are true, whatever things are honest, whatever things are just, whatever things are pure, whatever things are lovely, whatever things are of good report; if there be any virtue, and if there be any praise, think on these things" (Phil. 4:8).

Reject negative thinking. "Whatsoever is not of faith is sin" (Rom. 14:23).

There are sure to be some who will doubt your ability to achieve. They will point to all those times in the past when you had good intentions and failed. They will tell you it isn't worth it. A few may even try to sabotage your effort by bringing you gifts of your favorite foods. The calorie carrying kind. Others will have genuine compassion for you in the struggle, and will urge you to forget the whole thing so that you are not under such pressure.

Lovingly tune them out.

You have too much to lose by not losing. Your health, your happiness, and your future all get weighed each time you step on the scales.

Besides, you do not have to be fat. Remember, that mountain can be moved: " If ye have faith as a grain of mustard seed, ye shall say unto this mountain, 'Move from here to yonder place'; and it shall move; and nothing shall be impossible to you" (Matt 17:20).

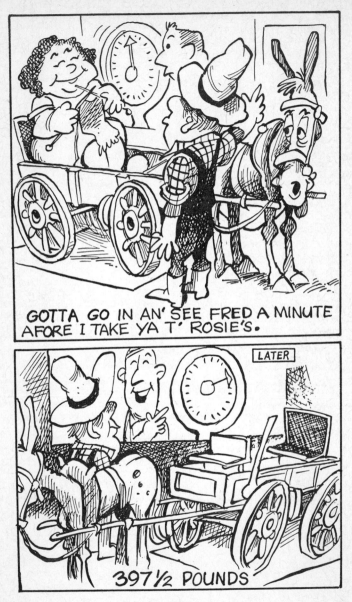

GOTTA GO IN AN' SEE FRED A MINUTE
AFORE I TAKE YA T' ROSIE'S.

LATER

397½ POUNDS

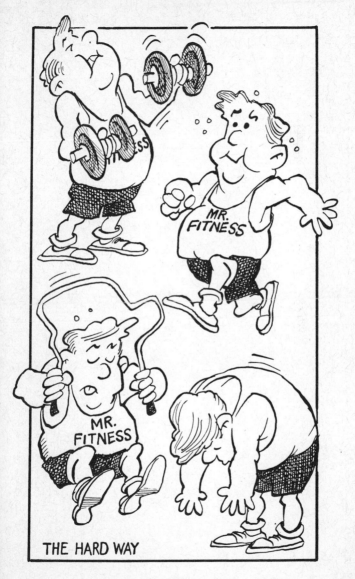

THE HARD WAY

"Then I claimed
the victory God
had given
to alcoholics
and drug addicts."

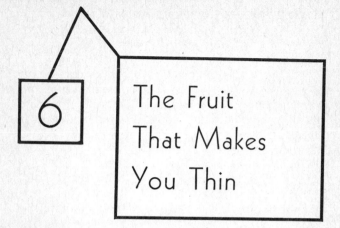

6 The Fruit That Makes You Thin

A young lady had her jaws wired together so she could eat no solid food. The wires remained till she had achieved her desired weight. Her method seems to have worked, but who wants to endure oral surgery every time pounds add up?

Dr. James Papsdorf, associate professor of psychology at the University of Michigan, is involved in a project to teach "self-management skills" to people who wish to lose weight. Dr. Papsdorf suggests the practice of giving up meaningful behavior if a person goes over the calorie count. This could be something as simple as giving up a favorite television program for a week or two.

Another approach is to bring home through the imagination the consequences of being overweight. Dr. Papsdorf urges his students to imagine themselves at their own funerals, or being bedridden with strokes, as a result of their overeating.

But should a Christian have to resort to such immature imaginings? There must be a better way.

The Holy Spirit—A Resource for Self-Control

We already know that the Christian's body is the temple of the Holy Spirit. This Divine Person within is not only a resident, but a resource. It is his purpose to reproduce the life of Jesus Christ in each of us. The Bible tells us what to expect when we allow that to happen: "But the fruit of the Spirit is love, joy, peace, long-suffering, gentleness, goodness, faith, meekness, self-control" (Gal. 5:22-23).

Now we know how Paul could confidently say: "But I keep under my body, and bring it into subjection" (1 Cor. 9:27). Since Paul was filled with the Holy Spirit, self-control was the inevitable result.

This is not new truth. We have long expected this in areas other than weight control. We have heard dynamic testimonies of deliverance from alcohol, tobacco, and drug addiction, temper, and other recognized sins. Somehow, intemperance in eating has escaped us. Rev. Pauley said it well.

Then I confessed to the Lord that it was just as much a sin for me to overeat as to smoke or drink. It was the beginning of victory for me when I called it a *sin*. I could have called it a shortcoming, but it was a real sin and it was wrong.

Then I claimed the victory that God had given to alcoholics and nicotine addicts. I did what I had asked teens to do several times—put God to the test. I said that either He was the God who can give me the victory over this sin or He was not the God that I thought He was, about whom I had preached through the years.

At that very moment God gave me the victory.[1]

---

[1] Pauley, *Mr. Before and After.*

So, the same power was sufficient for both Paul and Pauley. And their experience spans nearly two thousand years. It must be workable for you and me.

"All right," you say. "I'm convinced. I believe the Holy Spirit produces self-control. Why then don't I have it?"

If you do not have self-control, it is because you are not filled with the Holy Spirit. And that is commanded for every Christian: "And be not drunk with wine, in which is excess, but be filled with the Spirit" (Eph. 5:18).

Let us get it clear. The filling of the Holy Spirit is not an option for the Christian, it is obedience. How can you be filled?

You Must Stop Grieving the Holy Spirit

You may be surprised to know that God can be grieved. Yet, it is true. There are a number of texts in the Bible that reveal this.

Moses wrote that God was grieved over the wickedness that was on the earth before the flood: "And God saw that the wickedness of man was great in the earth, and that every imagination of the thoughts of his heart was only evil continually. And it repented the Lord that He had made man on the earth, and it grieved Him at his heart" (Gen. 6:5-6).

David reminded his people that God had been grieved with their forefathers when they grumbled in the wilderness, after their escape from Egypt: "Forty years long was I grieved with this generation, and said, 'It is a people that do err in their heart, and they have not known My ways'" (Ps. 95:10). Isaiah prophesied of the coming of our

Lord and called Him a "man of sorrows" and said that He would be "acquainted with grief" (53:3).

Jesus mourned over wayward Jerusalem (Luke 13:34-35), and wept at the grave of His friend Lazarus (John 11:35). Paul admonished the Christians at Ephesus "And grieve not the Holy Spirit of God, by whom ye are sealed unto the day of redemption. Let all bitterness, and wrath, and anger, and clamor, and evil speaking, be put away from you, with all malice; and be ye kind one to another, tender-hearted, forgiving one another, even as God for Christ's sake hath forgiven you" (Eph. 4:30-32).

Notice that all these sins that grieve the Holy Spirit have to do with your attitude toward others. You cannot be bitter toward others and be filled with the Holy Spirit. You cannot be angry with others and be filled with the Holy Spirit. You cannot gossip about others and be filled with the Holy Spirit. You cannot be filled with hatred and be filled with the Holy Spirit.

One would think that those converted to the crucified and forgiving Saviour would long since have laid aside such attitudes. But, sadly, it is not so. The eloquent DeWitt Talmadge observed:

There are in every community, and every church, watch dogs, who feel called upon to keep their eyes on others and growl. They are always the first to hear of anything wrong. Vultures are always the first to smell carrion. They are self-appointed detectives. I lay this down as a rule without exception, that those people who have the most faults themselves are the most merciless in their watching of others. From the scalp of head to soles of foot, they are full of jealousies, or hypercriticism. They spend their life hunting for muskrats and mud turtles, instead of hunting for rocky mountains and eagles, always for something mean instead of something grand. They look at their neighbors' imperfections through a telescope upside down.[2]

You cannot be one of that crowd and be filled with the Holy Spirit. And without the filling of the Spirit you cannot have the God-given self-control that you so badly need.

Your hate may determine your weight.

So, it is time to examine your life for things that grieve your Lord. Especially relating to others. As these wrong attitudes and actions are revealed to you, confess them immediately to Jesus. Then forsake and forget them: "If we confess our sins, He is faithful and just to forgive us our sins, and to cleanse us from all unrighteousness" (1 John 1:9).

You Must Stop Quenching the Holy Spirit

The Apostle Paul admonished, "Quench not the Spirit" (1 Thes. 5:19).

If we quench a fire, we stop it in its path. If we quench the Holy Spirit we halt His work in us. We stifle or suppress Him. When you quench the Holy Spirit you exalt your will above the will of God. To quench the Holy Spirit is to resist Him. It is going your own way when His leading is clear.

To avoid quenching the Holy Spirit, we need to know what He desires to do in our lives.

The Holy Spirit desires to comfort us (John 14:16).

The Holy Spirit desires to teach us (14:26).

---

[2] Walter B. Knight, *Knight's Master Book of New Illustrations,* (Grand Rapids, Mich.: William B. Eerdmans Publishing Company, 1956), p. 139.

The Holy Spirit desires to guide us into all truth (16:13).

The Holy Spirit desires to glorify Jesus (16:14).

The Holy Spirit desires to empower us (Acts 1:8).

The Holy Spirit desires to give us courage to witness (4:31-33).

The Holy Scripture desires to lead us (Rom. 8:14).

The Holy Spirit desires to bring forth fruit in us (Gal. 5:22-23).

The Holy Spirit desires to direct us in worship (Eph. 5:18-21).

In short, the Holy Spirit has a ministry in every area of your life. When you yield to Him you are in tune with the purpose of God for you. When you turn Him off you are quenching Him.

When you stop quenching the Holy Spirit you will find some wonderful things happening.

Your day will unfold as a part of His plan. You will see opportunities that you would have missed before.

You will be more aware of temptation and will be able to overcome it. Appetites will be tempered by His leading and wisdom. Whatever you eat or drink will be done to the glory of God.

His calming voice will comfort you when everything seems to be falling apart. Life's irritations will be recognized as experiences that enable you to be patient and longsuffering.

The needs of others will be brought to your attention and you will be refreshed in ministering to them. Having your own way will become less important. Allowing Christ to have His way in your life will receive priority.

You will find yourself responding to Bible instruction that you learned long ago, but had ignored in daily life.

Others will notice that you have an attitude of thanksgiving and praise, even on difficult days.

You will be constantly conscious of the presence of God.

So, stop tuning out the Holy Spirit. You cannot quench the Spirit and expect His fruit in your life. The moment you try to go it alone that elusive "self-control" will escape. You will be back on that old treadmill called "will power." From there it is but a short distance to gimmicks and failure again.

You Must Walk in the Spirit

Paul wrote to the Christians in Galatia: "This I say then, 'Walk in the Spirit, and ye shall not fulfill the lust of the flesh'" (Gal. 5:16).

Walking demonstrates faith.

Jesus told the man who had been sick of the palsy that he was to take up his bed and walk. That demanded faith. He had not been able to walk. The fact that he did get up and walk gave living evidence of his confidence in the power of Christ (Matt. 9:2-7).

Peter walked on the water to go to Jesus. That was a walk of faith. When Peter's faith faltered he began to sink (14:28-31). It was faith that made the miracle possible.

The person who walks in the Spirit has taken the filling of the Spirit by faith. As he moves through the day he expects the Holy Spirit to control him. And control is what the Spirit-filled life is all about. Does the Holy Spirit control your life? If not, you are controlled by your sinful nature.

The old nature. The old man. No wonder there have been so many disappointing experiences.

It is time to discover who sits on the throne of your life. Who is king? Lord? Master? The Bible teaches that either God rules over that kingdom called your life, or you live under sin's dominion. It's as simple as that. See how Paul explains this struggle and its solution to the Christians at Rome: "Likewise, reckon ye also yourselves to be dead indeed unto sin, but alive unto God through Jesus Christ, our Lord. Let not sin, therefore, reign in your mortal body, that ye should obey it in its lusts. Neither yield ye your members as instruments of unrighteousness unto sin, *but yield yourselves unto God, as those that are alive from the dead, and your members as instruments of righteousness unto God.* For sin shall not have dominion over you; for ye are not under the law but under grace" (Rom. 6:11-14).

Many years ago Dr. J. Wilbur Chapman wrote about his discovery of the Spirit-filled life. He said that he had been struggling for five years seeking the filling of the Holy Spirit. He shared the end of his search: "At last all my will was surrendered about everything. Then without emotion I said, 'My Father, I now claim from Thee the infilling of the Holy Spirit.'" [3]

Finally, Chapman realized that the object of his search had been within his grasp all the time. He stopped grieving and quenching the Holy Spirit. By faith, he claimed the filling of the Holy Spirit, and in that very moment, and by that act, began walking in the Spirit as a Spirit-filled man. He be-

---

[3] Knight, *Knight's Treasury of Illustrations,* p. 162.

came a man whose life demonstrated the fruit of the Spirit: love, joy, peace, long-suffering, gentleness, goodness, faith, meekness, self-control.

Self-control. How we need it! The Bible paints a tragic picture of the person who lacks it: "He that hath no rule over his own spirit is like a city that is broken down, and without walls" (Prov. 25:28).

Be filled with the Holy Spirit. That is your need. You will no longer be like a city that is broken down and without walls. Self-control will be yours. *It is the fruit that makes you thin.*

One further word. The filling of the Spirit is *not a one-time experience*. Unlike the baptism of the Spirit, the filling of the Holy Spirit is needed whenever we allow the old sin nature to assume control. You will not have to be told when that happens.

Thankfully, God's formula for filling is always available. Confess your sins (stop grieving the Spirit); surrender completely (stop quenching the Spirit); claim His filling by faith (walk in the Spirit); and all will be well again. His power and control will be yours so that you can become all that you ought to be.

By going
the second mile
you can lose
10 pounds a year.

eat, the only thing left is magic, so go ahead—whatever brand of magic you want." [3]

So you must become active to lose weight. And that is tough for many Americans. In his book *The New Aerobics*, Dr. Kenneth Cooper calls Americans the most inactive people in the world. An executive sits at his desk during most of his working hours. A student sits in a classroom all day and in a library at night. Millions of housewives sit through hours of soap operas in the afternoon and then relax with the family before the television during the evening. Salespersons kill hours between customers or spend much of their day in their automobiles getting to various business appointments. Gadgets and appliances help us get fat by opening our garage doors, washing our dishes, and even by assisting us in the steering and braking of our automobiles.

I wonder how many tons have been added to the frames of Americans by the installation of electric eye doors in public buildings.

Fat is sneaky. It slips up on us. And our modern way of life is loaded with opportunities for obesity. You can get fat without even trying. You may be buying pounds on the installment plan,—and paying fat finance charges.

How to Burn Calories
The housewife who used to expend 250 calories per hour doing her housework now has to burn up only 120 because of her "convenience" appliances. Meanwhile, unless she finds ways to exercise, her savings account of fat is increasing—with interest.

[3] Nancy Manser, "What, Snacking a Key to Losing All That Fat?" *Detroit News*, April 22, 1975

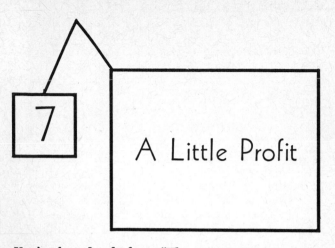

7 A Little Profit

You've heard it before: "The most important exercise in losing weight is pushing yourself away from the table."

This subtle half-truth implies that physical exercise isn't all that important. But it is.

I am married to a lady who keeps herself in shape. While it is very easy for her to put on pounds, she disciplines her body and stays within her chosen range of weight. For the past 10 years an exercise program has been a vital part of her success.

At some time during the morning, Pauline spends an hour alone in a locked room. For that hour the room is off limits to everyone, even to me. During that time she is exercising both soul and body. It is her time for devotions and calisthenics. Approximately one half of Pauline's special hour is given to physical exercise. In that time she goes through about 20 different types of exercises. They are the standard type that can be found in any good exercise book. Those 20 exercises require over 700 body movements—all of them consuming calories.

The Value of Exercise

Dr. O. Quentin Hyder has recommended this kind of program for everyone.

> Finally, don't forget to take plenty of exercise. This applies to everyone, obese or not. Our bodies transform food into energy. Energy that is not used up is stored as body fat. If we eat more than our bodies require for daily activities, we will get overweight. But if we exercise regularly, the excess available calories will be used up and we will not develop fat storage depots around the abdomen and hips. Exercise should not be thought of as something painful done to control weight and keep the body fit. It can also be fun. Calisthenics at home are convenient and burn up 500 unwanted calories per hour if done with sustained effort.[1]

Some Christians quote the Bible as a cop-out on any exercise program. Their favorite verse is 1 Timothy 4:8: "For bodily exercise profiteth little, but godliness is profitable unto all things, having the promise of the life that now is, and of that which is to come."

At first reading one would think that Paul was scorning physical exercise. A closer study of the verse, however, reveals that he was simply comparing the importance of physical exercise to that of spiritual. Naturally, spiritual gains are more important than physical, though in some cases they are closely related.

[1] Hyder, *The Christian's Handbook of Psychiatry*. Used by permission.

Another version renders the verse this way: "Fo physical training has some value in it . . ." (AMP)

The Bible teaches, then, that there is value in physical exercise. It is not to be compared with such things as prayer and Bible study, but, nevertheless, it has value.

It certainly has value in controlling weight. There's no doubt about it. Here's why: *Activity uses up calories!* It's as simple as that.

Common sense then brings you to a conclusion: *You can control calories by both diet and exercise.* If you neglect either, your effort to control your weight is more likely to fail.

Dr. Jean Mayer urges losers to balance both sides of their calorie expense account. He warns those who would spend calories:

> The final widespread fallacy that stands in the way of successful dieting is the belief that food intake alone determines how much you gain or lose. In fact, like your bank balance, your weight depends on how much you take out as well as how much you put in. It is far more difficult to reduce if the only muscles you ever move are the chewing muscles. It is considerably easier and far more healthful to lose weight by a combination of calorie reduction and exercise than it is by calorie cutting alone.[2]

Dr. Lawrence Power, professor of internal medicine at Wayne State University, put it bluntly. He said: "There is no way you can take on calories in excess of your need without them accumulating. If you're not going to exercise and watch what you

[2] Dr. Jean Mayer, "Secrets of Making Your Diet Work" as condensed in the June 1972 *Reader's Digest*. Reprinted with permission of *Family Health* Magazine, November 1971 ©. All rights reserved.

A typist using a manual typewriter burns about 88 calories each hour. If her boss wants to please her and buys her an electric typewriter she will cut her calorie need to 73 calories hourly. At the end of the first week with her new typewriter she will have stored 450 calories, and if she doesn't cut her intake of food or increase her exercise she will gain an extra pound every two months. If she stays at the job for five years she will have added 30 pounds.

If you are serious, then, about losing weight, you must fight fire with fire. You must begin to look for opportunities to exercise. And they are all about us.

While dining at a parsonage, the pastor's wife told me of her struggle to lose weight. I thought the least I could do, as a guest, was to make a helpful suggestion on this touchy subject. I suggested that the pastor might help his wife lose weight. They seemed interested, so I ventured further. I advised the pastor to keep reminding his wife that every household chore could be another opportunity for her in her effort to become slim again.

She was caring for two small children besides her own, so I was sure there would be many occasions for her to do extra work around the house. I urged her husband to enthusiastically point out this great privilege to his wife every time the children spilled their food or tracked dirt across a clean floor.

"I'd kill him," she said.

And I hear a thousand tired young mothers sighing, "Amen!"

Of course few husbands would dare follow the rash advice I gave the preacher that day. Yet, there was sound instruction in this tongue-in-cheek dining room direction. There are many opportunities for exercise in our daily routine. We just need to take advantage of them.

For many years I have jogged from parking spots to appointments. This practice not only helps me keep in shape but increases my efficiency on the job. It makes better use of my time. Seeing a man with a Bible run across a hospital parking lot toward the hospital may be startling to onlookers. If they conclude that someone is dying, they are wrong. It is just someone living.

You may need to eliminate an extension telephone. The telephone company boasts that one extension phone saves the average person 76 miles of walking in a year. That saving of activity will add approximately two pounds in weight that you don't need. When it comes to extra phones, you're better off to stick with long distance.

Since our children are all grown we are beginning to look for a smaller home. One of my wife's requirements is stairs—lots of them. She knows the value of that added exercise and doesn't want to lose that by moving to a smaller house. Stair climbing expends ten calories a minute—that's two and a half times as much as walking. Think of the opportunities you have lost by calling up to your children instead of climbing the stairs to deliver a message. Think of all the times you have tossed dirty clothes down the basement stairs and have missed the advantage of taking them down and walking up the stairs again.

Stop looking for the parking place closest to your destination. You'll probably save time when you eliminate going around the same block a half dozen times, and the longer walk will fit into your daily exercise program.

Eliminate elevators and escalators whenever possible. That is, of course, if your general health allows it, a rule that should apply to any exercise experience.

Go for a walk with your wife or husband. Your marriage may need the romance and your body definitely needs the exercise.

Walking is largely neglected in our mobile society. Dr. Vance Havner says that walking is his only "un-American activity." Yet it is extremely healthful and a great exercise. In addition, it is a natural tranquilizer.

The American Medical Association says that a walk of just an extra mile each day for 36 days provides a pleasant way of shedding an extra pound of fat. The extra mile is defined as just that—a mile of walking in addition to the amount you have been doing. So, by going the second mile you can lose ten pounds a year. Providing, of course, that you do not increase your calorie intake as you increase your exercise.

Sports are good exercise. Team sports are fine when children are of school age, but not too valuable later. More enduring activities such as tennis and swimming can be shared by the whole family.

Bicycling has caught on for all ages and is another energy user that can involve group exercise and fun.

On the following page is a list of daily responsibilities and recreational activities showing the calories used per hour in each. How many of these are a part of your average day?

	Approximate calories used per hour for:	
	130 lb. person	175 lb. person
Activity		
Making bed	247	332
Bicycling—fast	520	700
Calisthenics	247	332
Driving car	117	157
Dishwashing	117	157
Eating	91	122
Football	468	630
Gardening	299	402
Golf	156	210
Ironing	130	175
Mopping floors	130	175
Office work	104	140
Painting—household	156	210
Ping-pong	325	437
Resting	65	88
Rowing	650	875
Sewing (machine)	91	122
Singing	117	157
Skiing	676	910
Sweeping—broom	143	192
Swimming	533	717
Tennis	364	490
Vacuuming	286	385
Walking fast	260	350
Writing	91	122
Running	481	647

Be alert for opportunities for any extra motion or action that will use calories. This produces a delightful life-style. Rather than pouting about having to do something extra, the Christian dieter constantly looks for something more to do.

Bertha is 68 years old and her husband, Art, is 75. Bertha followed the Lose Weight the Bible Way course closely and began losing weight so quickly that I became concerned about her. She had been troubled with some health problems in the past and I was afraid that she might be overdoing. One day I stopped her in the foyer of the church and expressed my fears to her. I was about to urge her to slow down a bit when she stopped me short. "I've talked this over with my doctor," she said, "and he's really pleased with my weight loss." At that point Art spoke up and said, "But I'm sure having trouble getting used to Bertha opening every door for me." We laughed together and they went on their way, with Art rejoicing and Bertha reducing.

Yes, bodily exercise is of some value. According to Dr. George V. Mann, it is the most underrated aspect of conquering obesity. If you've been trying to lose weight without increasing daily exercise, recognizing this important fact may be one key to future success.

Eating with all
your heart
is the satisfying
experience of focusing
on the quality of food.

8 Take The Plunge

It must be clear by now that losing weight involves a significant change in life-style. This is no two-week wonder that melts off pounds, only to pick them up again a fortnight later. It is, instead, a different way of life.

Review the formula:

A. You will *care* for God's temple.
B. You will *conquer* depression through prayer and the application of God's Word.
C. You will *confront* your enemy, Satan, and see him defeated through your victorious Saviour.
D. You will have *confidence* that God will enable you to achieve your goal.
E. You will have *control* through the Holy Spirit.
F. You will *capture* opportunities for exercise.

There is another important ingredient. It might be called "plunging into life." This approach to daily duty is a delightful mixture of Christian optimism and enthusiasm. Biblically, it is the way to live. "And whatever you do, do it heartily, as to the Lord, and not unto men" (Col. 3:23). "Whatsoever thy hand findeth to do, do it with thy might" (Ecc. 9:10).

What you do is important. How you do it may be even more important.

The Example of Jesus

Jesus was the greatest example of one who gave Himself completely to every task He did. Wherever He went the mundane was made miraculous. Everyday contacts were recognized as divine opportunities. Common sights became teaching tools: the sower, the fig tree, the vine and the branches.

He gave His best to every situation.

Invite Him to a wedding feast and when the wine runs out He will produce better wine than the ruler of the feast has ever tasted (John 2:1-10).

Send Him through Samaria, hungry, thirsty, and tired, and He will find a troubled woman beside a well. He addresses Himself to her need. His fatigue is not a factor now, nor are His needs for food and water. It is her thirst of soul that counts. Before she leaves He will give her living water so that she will never thirst again. And to the amazement of His disciples, He will neither rest nor eat until He has ministered to her many friends who have come out from the city to hear and to believe (4:4-43).

Give Him a congregation of 5,000. Let the day draw to a close. Supply Him with five barley loaves and two small fishes, and He will feed the multitude and there will be 12 baskets of leftovers (6:1-13).

Call Him at the death of Lazarus. Watch Him

weep beside the tomb. Hear Him call Lazarus forth from the grave. Share the joy of Mary and Martha as they receive their brother alive again, but remember that this journey to Bethany will end at the cross. He knew that, but still responded to their call (11:1-44).

Follow Him into the Garden of Gethsemane. Witness His agony as He prays so earnestly that His sweat falls like drops of blood from His brow, and understand that this scene measures the intensity of His life and purpose (Luke 22:39-44).

Place Him on a cross. Pound nails through His hands and feet. Crown Him with thorns. Let the crowds spit on Him and mock Him. Watch while Roman soldiers gamble for His garments beneath the cross. Crucify a thief on either side of Him. By now you will have concluded that there is nothing more He can give, but if you listen carefully you will hear Him guarantee Paradise to a dying thief. He made the most of the moment. He lived and died with all His heart.

Other Biblical Examples

With such an example, it is not surprising to find the New Testament writers calling for *fervency* in the Christian life. Paul begged the Christians in Rome to be fervent in spirit: "Not slothful in business; fervent in spirit, serving the Lord" (Rom. 12:11).

Peter asked his readers to be fervent in their love for each other. "Seeing that ye have purified your souls in obeying the truth through the Spirit unto unfeigned love of the brethren, see that ye love one another with a pure heart fervently" (1 Peter 1:22). James urged fervency in prayer.

"The effectual fervent prayer of a righteous man availeth much" (James 5:16).

And those early Christians were fervent! The word was out that they had "turned the world upside down" (Acts 17:6). You and I have the Gospel today because they gave themselves to the task with all their hearts.

There are biblical grounds for living intensely. The message is vital, the time is short, and the need is great. The task is overwhelming. If for no other reason, the Christian should attack all projects energetically so that he will have additional opportunities and contacts to carry the message of Christ to others.

Bible heroes were men and women of action.

Consider Moses facing Pharaoh, producing plagues, dividing the sea, and leading that great multitude through the wilderness. And all this after he was 80 years old. Some senior citizen!

Think of Joshua taking over after the death of Moses. There was the flooded Jordan to cross and Canaan to conquer. He trembled at first, but finally threw himself into the task and emerged triumphant. He saw the walls of Jericho fall and the land divided to his people, as God had promised. One day he became so immersed in his work that he begged God for more daylight so he could finish the job. God granted his request. The Bible says: "So the sun stood still in the midst of heaven, and hastened not to go down about a whole day. And there was no day like that before it or after it" (Josh. 10:13-14).

The Book of Proverbs gives a description of a "virtuous woman." She is a busy woman, to say the least. She appears to be industrious, compassionate, and totally involved in life. She is a giving person who is serving others from morning until night. (See Proverbs 31:10-31.)

A study of the Book of Psalms reveals that David was a man who lived 60 minutes of every hour. His moods and experiences take one from the tops of the mountains to the depths of the valleys and back again. Sometimes he was sobbing, sometimes singing. There were times of triumph and times when he seemed to be hanging on for dear life. But one thing is sure: David tackled both duty and devotion with his whole heart. He declares, "Blessed are the undefiled in the way, who walk in the law of the Lord. Blessed are they that keep *his* testimonies, and that seek Him with the whole heart. With my whole heart have I sought Thee; oh, let me not wander from Thy commandments" (Ps. 119:1-2, 10).

Paul pictured himself as an athlete. Outwardly, he didn't really fit that image—he wouldn't have qualified for the Olympics. But he seized each day for his Saviour. He called upon his hearers to make the best use of every moment. "Redeeming the time," he called it (Eph. 5:18). He must have practiced what he preached, for no man could have coasted through life and equaled Paul's accomplishments. What was the dynamic that drove him on? Let Paul tell it: "I press toward the mark for the prize of the high calling of God in Christ Jesus" (Phil. 3:14).

The Bible commends an active life; it condemns idleness.

Intense Christian Living
A number of years ago I went through a brief

period of struggling with laziness. It was not brief because of any great qualities I possess, but because of the battering I received in my personal devotions at that time. I was then going through the Book of Proverbs, hazardous reading for anyone who wishes to loaf. These are some of the verses that ended my indolence. "How long wilt thou sleep, O sluggard? When wilt thou arise out of thy sleep? Yet a little sleep, a little slumber, a little folding of the hands to sleep, so shall thy poverty come like one that traveleth, and thy want like an armed man" (6:9-11). "The slothful man saith, There is a lion outside; I shall be slain in the streets" (22:13). "As the door turneth upon his hinges, so doth the slothful upon his bed. The slothful hideth his hand in his dish; it grieveth him to bring it again to his mouth" (26:14-15).

I couldn't stand up (or lie down) under that punishment; now I read the Book of Proverbs every time I feel the need of another push.

The Christian life is to be an active and intense life. Whatever we do should get our best effort. Jesus Christ has set the example.

What does that have to do with losing weight? Potentially, a great deal. Common sense tells us that extra effort uses more energy and thus helps remove fat, but is that a proper motive for enthusiastic Christian service? I think not. That would be placing the cart before the horse. It would produce a spurt of activity for a time, till the weight was normal, and then the old lifestyle would return. I also question the value of such self-serving service. Would it really be effective? How would it stand up at the judgment seat of Christ? Poorly, I'm afraid.

The proper approach is from the other direction. We must serve the Lord with all our hearts because we love Him. We must plunge into life because He has set the example. We must give Him our best because He deserves it. We must seize opportunities because He has placed them in our way.

The rewards we receive from true dedication and service will be ours at His return. "And, behold, I come quickly and my reward is with Me, to give every man according as his work shall be" (Rev. 22:12).

Meanwhile, back on Planet Earth, there are some wonderful fringe benefits that accompany consecrated Christian service. There is the satisfaction of obeying God's Word. There is the joy of seeing others influenced toward God by our lives. There are the advantages given our body, God's temple, through the discipline, control, and activity of Christian living. Not the least of those advantages is the loss of unwanted pounds.

The Fat Fringe Benefit

If you get a spring in your step, and you do not increase your intake of food, it must make a difference in your weight. Recently, at the University of California, Irvine, Dr. Grant Gwinup studied a group of overweight women who for a year took a *brisk* walk for half an hour each day. They lost an average of 22 pounds each from brisk walking alone (the range of loss was from 10 to 38 pounds). Their diets were not restricted during this time, and some even ate more because of the increased appetite after exercise.

If you eat one chicken T.V. dinner containing 542 calories, and lie down, it will take you 217 minutes to use up those calories. If you take a walk, the energy will be burned up in 104 minutes. If you ride a bicycle it will take 66 minutes. If you run, your caloric energy will be entirely used in less than half an hour (28 minutes).

A boiled egg contains about 77 calories. It will supply caloric energy for approximately one hour if you are lying down. Walking will exhaust the energy from your egg in 15 minutes. The more brisk your walk the faster your calories will be used up, and if you break into a run that egg will last only four minutes.

Roast beef with gravy, containing 430 calories, will have its caloric energy consumed in 83 minutes of walking. The extra exertion of swimming will burn those same calories in 38 minutes, and running will use them in 22 minutes. I do not mean to encourage running or swimming immediately after eating, but the message ought to be getting through. A new zest for life that adds activity will cause you to lose weight, unless you eat more and cancel out your gains.

Rise earlier.

Attempt more.

Squeeze the life out of every second.

Savor life.

Come alive.

Change your attitude about eating. Make mealtime more than fill-up-time. Enjoy the people around your table. Delight in each delicious mouthful. Determine to make your meal last longer without eating more. Take smaller bites so that you will not finish so quickly. Generally, people who eat slowly have fewer weight problems. That is because the stomach needs time to notify the brain that sufficient food has arrived. Eating with all your heart is the satisfying experience of focusing on the quality, rather than the quantity, of food.

There is another dimension to plunging into life. It involves the conquering of those fears that have kept you from doing the things you have really wanted to do. Fears that may have prevented you from doing God's will.

You have a creative heart and mind, but you do not create.

You would like to attempt a number of things but you hold back because you are afraid of failure. You would rather be safe than embarrassed. But adventure or creativity—whichever word you like best—always involves risks. It involves a decision; it is purposive; it is an expression of yourself. Usually it involves others. It stretches you, so that you end up being more than you ever thought you could be. It adds the special flavor to life that makes you feel that you have a secret with God.

At this point you may be thinking of the composition of an exciting piece of music, or a new harmonic arrangement, or a painting, or a poem. And you've already said, 'I can't do that.' Then don't do that. Find something your own size. It may be learning how to knit; it may be flying a kite on a hillside with your son and getting the tail the right length so that it will soar out of sight in the blue, blue of the spring sky.

Creativity is taking the stuff of life that exists and shaping it. It is to be for the moment a spark of communication between God and man, reflecting some small piece of His creative nature.[1]

[1] From *Ms. Means Myself* by Gladys Hunt. Copyright © 1973 by Gladys Hunt and is used by permission.

Take the risk. Plunge into life and taste its abundance. It will help to *shape up* your future and fulfill the purpose of Jesus Christ in you. He said, "I am come that they might have life, and that they might have it more abundantly" (John 10:10).

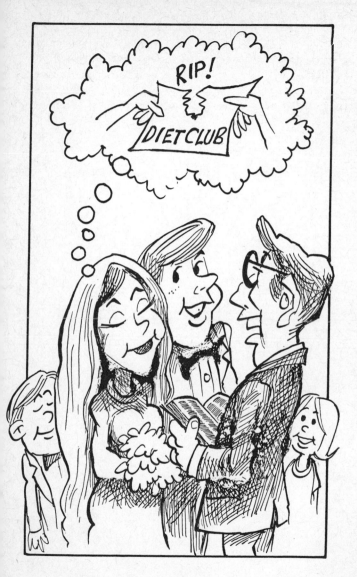

Find your function
in the body
of Christ
and perform
it with enthusiasm.

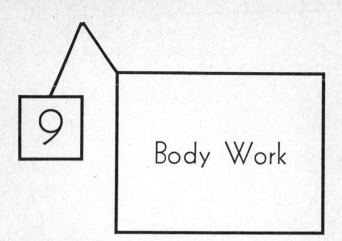

9

Body Work

Christians have the advantage in any undertaking that involves discipline of the body and mind.

The reason? Their resources.

When Larry came into my office it was evident that something good had happened in his life. His wife had called earlier in the week to make the appointment. He had contacted her from across the state, where he was working, and asked her to put away all the ashtrays and to make an appointment with me.

I knew, of course, that this meeting had something to do with Larry's desire to quit smoking. I was to learn, however, that his victory over tobacco was only the tip of the iceberg.

Larry's grandfather had been a minister of the Gospel and had led him to Christ when he was a child. Larry had wrestled with temptation in his teen years and had gone down in defeat a number of times. As the years passed, habits accumulated that held him in their grip. By observing his life you would not have known that he was a Christian. Then came that unforgettable night in a motel room in Muskegon, Michigan.

Larry had finished his work for the day as a railroad police safety instructor and had decided to stop by a local bar to relax. When he left the bar he was intoxicated.

After arriving at his motel room, Larry fell asleep, awaking at about nine that evening. He was surprised to find his head clear. He was completely sober, and a Bible verse his grandfather had taught him long ago was running through his mind. It was Psalm 119:11: "Thy word have I hid in mine heart, that I might not sin against Thee." He tried to shake it off. He smoked a cigarette. It didn't help. He tried watching television to divert his mind, but still that verse kept haunting him.

Finally at two in the morning, Larry looked upward and cried, "All right, You've won!" He went on in his prayer confessing his sins and dedicating his life to Jesus Christ. He is now free from both tobacco and alcohol. Even his reading habits have changed. The magazines that used to feed his lust are not a part of his life anymore. He is a liberated man.

Factors in Fulfillment

What were the factors that brought about Larry's new-found freedom? They were the Holy Spirit, the Bible, faith, and prayer. During the years that Larry paid little attention to these dynamic forces, he was a defeated person. The moment he surrendered his will and began to use the resources God had given him, he became a conqueror.

Many Christians have an experience similar to

Larry's in background. The details vary, but the struggle with temptation and the ultimate victory are much alike. There is both a triumph and a tragedy about too many of these experiences. It is wonderful when a Christian discovers that God has equipped him with power to overcome all temptation. The moment of victory is sweet, and the resulting testimony is often effective in the lives of others. If, however, he lives the rest of his life in the shadow of that one experience and majors henceforth on the things that he *does not do*, it is tragic.

It is a sad fact that many have come to identify Christians by observing those things that they *do not do*. Some negatives are needed in the Christian life, but it is a mistake to feel that in abstaining from a half dozen worldly practices we have fulfilled our Christian obligation.

It was exciting for me to listen to Larry as he described his deliverance from dependence, but it has been more thrilling to see him in action serving his Lord.

The Battle Isn't Over Yet

Many Christians exercise only a portion of their potential and fulfill only a fraction of their purpose in life. They have learned the secrets of discipline and control but have stopped there. Practically speaking, they have relaxed after winning the first few battles. They ease through life as if the war was over.

Double trouble occurs when activities involving food take the place of former diversions. Christians often feel they can substitute calories for carnality. Actually, both cater to the flesh.

Nor is inactivity spiritual. We may long for some quiet haven, but God seems always to have called busy men into His service. Moses was tending sheep. David was caring for his father's flocks while his brothers were being viewed for kingly qualities. Elisha was plowing with twelve yoke of oxen. Peter was fishing, and that was his daily work. It ought to be clear that the new birth ushers in a more active life. God has work for you to do.

The Christian life described in the Bible is both abundant and active; it is disciplined and dynamic.

There is a commission to obey and a world to win. Jesus said: "Go ye, therefore, and teach all nations, baptizing them in the name of the Father, and of the Son, and of the Holy Spirit" (Matt. 28:19). "But ye shall receive power, after that the Holy Spirit is come upon you; and ye shall be witnesses unto Me both in Jerusalem, and in all Judea, and in Samaria, and unto the uttermost part of the earth" (Acts 1:8).

A look at the Early Church reveals an involved and active group of people. Even in persecution they were about their Lord's business. "Therefore, they that were scattered abroad went everywhere preaching the word" (Acts 8:4).

Actually, the church has often thrived under persecution while becoming lazy and ineffective during times of prosperity. Perhaps that is because all the saints are activated under pressure.

Today's church is often afflicted by the "spectator syndrome." The saints sit and soak while the pastor does most of the ministering. But that is simply not God's plan for His people. Here's the plan: "And He gave some, apostles; and some prophets; and some, evangelists; and some pastors and teachers; for the perfecting of the saints for the work of the ministry for the edifying of the body of Christ" (Eph. 4:11-12).

Every Christian is to be ministering.

Your Part of the Body

The purpose of your ministry is to build up the body of Christ, which is made up of all Christians everywhere.

As a part of the body of Christ you are flesh and bone of the living organism through which our Lord works in this world:

> For as the body is one, and hath many members, and all the members of that one body, being many, are one body, so also is Christ. For by one Spirit were we all baptized into one body, whether we be Jews or Greeks, whether we be bond or free; and have all made to drink unto one Spirit. For the body is not one member, but many (1 Cor. 12:12-14).

We all know that any part of our body that is not performing its normal function finally becomes weak and useless. A similar condition develops in the body of Christ. You must stay active to remain healthy.

Regardless of your ability or appearance, you are a very important member of the body of Christ:

> If the foot shall say, Because I am not the hand, I am not of the body; is it, therefore, not of the body? And if the ear shall say, Because I am not the eye, I am not of the body; is it, therefore, not of the body? If the whole body were an eye, where were the hearing? If the whole body were hearing, where were the smelling? But now God hath set the members, every one of them, in the body, as it hath pleased Him (12:15-18).

There is no excuse for inactivity. God has given you everything necessary to perform your work in this world. Whether you are ministering to the needs of other Christians or busy in the evangelization of your community or the world, you can do the task God intends for you to do. Remember you have been placed in the body "as it hath pleased Him."

So, get busy for Christ!

Begin where you are and with what you have.

Visit someone who is sick and pray for him.

Take some food to a needy brother or sister.

Join the choir.

Volunteer to teach a Sunday School class.

Shock your pastor by showing up for visitation.

Offer to help in the church office.

Distribute tracts throughout your neighborhood.

Encourage someone who is down.

Spend an hour helping a widow.

Invite the youth of your church to your home for one of their meetings.

If you really want to serve, opportunities will open all around you. You'll be blessed in your ministry and that wonderful fringe benefit will accompany the blessing, for you will be using up calories with every move you make.

Want to be a slim saint? Then find your function in the body of Christ and perform it with enthusiasm.

Another exciting dimension to our responsibility as a part of the body of Christ involves the gifts God has given to enable us to be effective. Paul taught the Christians in Rome about their gifts and the importance of using them. He explained:

For as we have many members in one body, and all

members have not the same office, so we, being many, are one body in Christ, and every one members one of another. Having gifts differing according to the grace that is given to us, whether prophecy, let us prophesy according to the proportion of faith; or ministry, let us wait on our ministering; or he that teacheth, on teaching, or he that exhorteth, on exhortation; he that giveth, let him do it with liberality; he that ruleth, with diligence; he that showeth mercy, with cheerfulness" (Rom. 12:3-8).

It doesn't take a great deal of discernment to notice that Christians do not all have the same gifts. Much harm has been done in the body of Christ by some members trying to copy the ministry of others rather than using their own gifts. The consequence is often frustration and fruitlessness.

When I was a boy I lived on a grain and dairy farm. The soil was heavy and quite fertile and usually produced fine crops. Even when the summer was very dry, our fields looked comparatively green and healthy because the soil retained moisture so well. A few miles west of our farm, nearer Lake Michigan, the soil was light and sandy. There the farming was very poor, especially during a dry season. Many summers the corn browned and curled, a discouraging sight for the struggling farmers who lived there.

Today, however, this area is a prosperous farming community, which ships its produce to many distant places. It is one of the most productive blueberry areas in the United States.

The secret of this agricultural success story was simply planting a crop for which the soil and climate were well-suited. And that is a good lesson for life.

If you want to be effective as a member of the body of Christ, serve with the gifts that God has given to you. Stop trying to be someone else. Diversity is part of God's wonderful plan.

Knowing Your Gifts

"But how do I know which gifts I possess?" you ask. You're fortunate. A number of good books have been written to answer your question. I especially recommend: *19 Gifts of the Spirit* by Leslie Flynn (Victor Books, Wheaton, Ill.), *Body Life* by Ray C. Stedman (Regal Books, Glendale, Calif.), and *Tongues in a Biblical Perspective* by Charles R. Smith (B.M.H. Books, Winona Lake, Ind.).

While not attempting to be as complete as the studies listed above, I will make a few suggestions that may help you in discovering your gifts.

First, read everything you can find in the Bible about spiritual gifts and gifts to the church. The major portions are Romans 12, 1 Corinthians 12—14, and Ephesians 4.

Second, begin obeying the commands of the Bible that have to do with service.

Even if we thought we had no gifts, or were unaware of our responsibility to discover and develop our gifts, we do possess hundreds of New Testament commands which operate in the area of gifts. Everyone, without possessing the following gifts, is enjoined to evangelize, exhort, show mercy, and help. As we begin to obey in these or other spheres, the Holy Spirit gradually unveils certain gifts. So we should get busy in Christian service.[1]

---

[1] Leslie Flynn, *19 Gifts of the Spirit*, Wheaton, Ill.: Victor Books, 1974, p. 194.

Third, look for your gifts in those areas of life and service in which you are most comfortable.

A dedicated Christian lady once came to me greatly distressed about finding her gifts. She had been teaching children successfully for years and loved it, but had recently been advised that her satisfaction or success had nothing to do with whether or not she was using her gifts that God had given her. She wanted to continue her work with children, but was willing to stop that ministry in order to search for her gifts. I helped her see that one of her gifts was teaching, and that God had confirmed this in the results and joy that He had given in that ministry. She left my office happy in the thought that she had been using her gifts all along. She and the children have been benefiting from that obvious discovery for more than ten years.

Fourth, accept opportunities to do things that you have not done before. You may discover gifts that are dormant because you have never used them.

"How would you like to preach tonight?" I once asked a layman, somewhat facetiously. His answer surprised me. "I'll be glad to. I have promised the Lord that I will accept every opportunity He sends my way." He is now a missionary in South America.

A young man was asked to teach an adult Bible class in Sunday School. He didn't feel qualified, but accepted. Shortly after he began teaching, a new pastor came to his church and noticed immediately his gift of teaching. The class grew and the young man developed spiritually. Today he is a successful pastor.

Fifth, be open to observations by other Christians concerning your spiritual gifts. Flynn noted:

> As we are doing Christian service in obedience to
> the commands of Christ, others may see a gift in
> us long before we ourselves are aware of it. In fact,
> the joy and preoccupation of ministry may make us
> temporarily oblivious to the special abilities which
> the Spirit has given us. A vital duty of Christians
> is to encourage fellow believers when they observe
> a gift.[2]

On this point, however, we must be prayerful.
Jesus said that a prophet is not always honored in
his own country, and that truth has often held back
proper recognition in the home church of the
gifted person.

On the other side is the enthusiasm of those who
love us. Well-meaning friends or relatives may
come on strong with words of praise while being
blind to our weaknesses. Their actions or reactions
may not be valid because they are based wholly
on their feelings for us.

Somewhere between these extremes the wise believer can find help from others in discovering his
gifts.

As a Christian, then, you are both equipped for
action and challenged to the ultimate of your potential. Few saints serve sufficiently. As a result,
the world remains unevangelized and the Body of
Christ suffers.

You may never have considered how much you
can lose, both physically and spiritually, by not
fulfilling your role as a member of His body. Consider it now. The Bible commands it; the times
demand it: "Wherefore, he saith, Awake thou that

---

[2] Flynn, *19 Gifts of the Spirit,* p. 201.

sleepest, . . . and Christ shall give thee light. See, then, that ye walk circumspectly, not as fools but as wise, redeeming the time, because the days are evil. Wherefore, be ye not unwise but understanding what the will of the Lord is" (Eph. 5:14-17).

It is interesting, yet true, that the child of God who makes the best use of his time and talents to build up the body of Christ will be so active that his own body will profit from the Christian lifestyle. If his appetite is controlled by the Holy Spirit, excess weight will be used up.

What a satisfying way to live—and lose!

Has your spouse
mentioned
a "spare tire"
when automobiles are not the
topic of conversation?

For Married Losers

Married losers have a lot to gain:
  A longer life together
  Improved health
  Fewer emotional hang-ups
  A better love life.

As a pastor, I am selective about the couples I marry, and I spend considerable time with them. My counseling sessions contain biblical instruction and life experiences that I expect will help mold a lasting love relationship. Yet, in spite of my efforts, some of these marriages fail.

Marriage is under fire these days. The pressures of modern society and the loosing of old and established mores have taken a deadly toll on many homes that started well. Even Christian homes are feeling the strain, and some are breaking up.

Christian married couples should have everything going for them. Bible reading and prayer in the home ought to be a daily experience. Involvement in the work of Christ through the local church ought to add inspiration and purpose to life. The ministry of God's Word in the public worship services ought to aid in building upon a solid foundation. But these alone will not guarantee a good marriage.

Good health and emotional well-being are also important factors in a meaningful marriage. Since it has already been shown that an overweight condition affects both of these areas of life, it makes sense to know what to do when fat invades the family.

Perhaps you are not sure whether weight is a problem in your home. Here are ten thought stimulators to help you decide:

1. Can you still wear your wedding gown?
2. Is your tuxedo size the same as on your wedding day?
3. Do you fit as comfortably in each other's arms now as then?
4. Does your wedding ring fit?
5. Is fat threatening fidelity?
6. Has your husband told you that he now has more wife to love?
7. Has your wife mentioned a "spare tire" when automobiles are not the topic of conversation?
8. Has she inquired about the status of your life insurance?
9. Would (could) he still carry you over the threshold?
10. Did you get a Weight Watcher's membership for Christmas?

If you feel like pleading the fifth amendment to any of the above questions, it's time to get serious about weight control.

Reasons for Heavy Marrieds

That once-perfect form may have been altered by a change in eating habits. Your diet before marriage may have been healthful and relatively free from calorie-rich desserts and delicacies. It was your husband's demand to come across with hot mince pie, strawberry shortcake, and other goodies that caused your problem. He said that he had been working hard all day and needed plenty of home-cooked food like his mother used to make. You produced, and now you both show it.

Or it may have been those calorie-laden creations of your new bride. Your better judgment told you to take it easy, but she seemed hurt when you didn't eat everything she had prepared, so you co-operated. Today, you are living proof of your co-operation.

Some heavy marrieds are the result of the oh-well-I've-got-him-now attitude. Before the wedding, appearance was important. After, it didn't matter. Caution was thrown to the winds. The prize was already won. Captive. The problem with this attitude is that some captives seek freedom. It's a dangerous way to live.

Sometimes pounds are added by the stress of new responsibilities brought by married life. Concern over unpaid bills, disobedient children, marital strife, and other pressures have sent many husbands and wives to the refrigerator in the late hours of the night. The catch in this kind of diversion is that it only adds another problem.

Pregnancies produce pounds. With each child you may have added pounds. Excusable? Perhaps a few times, but not forever. Mothers have an added obligation to slim down for their children's sake.

Some mates have a hard time pinpointing the reason for their increased weight. It just slipped up on them. They were not aware of any fast gain but can hardly believe their eyes when they look at their wedding pictures. "Is that us?" In this case, advancing age may have been the culprit. Fewer calories are required as we reach maturity. Yet, food intake is often unchanged. The result is predictable.

Then, of course, there are those who were overweight when they were married. "He knew I was fat when he married me." Does that mean you should go on punishing yourself? Think about it. There's a better way to live.

Helping Each Other

In one way, married people who are trying to lose weight have an advantage over singles. They can help one another. That's biblical: "And the Lord God said, It is not good that the man should be alone; I will make him an help fit for him" (Gen. 2:18).

The wise wife will not prepare fattening foods for her overweight husband. She will make a special effort to prepare delicious low-calorie dishes. She will search for new recipes that provide variety without adding pounds. Desserts will be few. Temptation removed. She will consider his effort to shed pounds a matter of life and death. And it is.

Likewise, the helpful husband will encourage his wife when she is making an effort to regain her former figure. He will not ridicule her or sabotage her diet. He will not bring home sweet treats, and he will refrain from taking her to expensive restaurants where the rich foods seem irresistible.

The Christian couple will remember that all temptation can be overcome: "There hath no temptation taken you but such as is common to man; but God is faithful, who will not permit you to be tempted above that ye are able, but will with the temptation, also make the way to escape, that ye may be able to bear it" (1 Cor. 10:13).

It will also be valuable to let the heavier mate get the most action. This will be difficult for some, especially husbands. Our culture has taught us that the man is to make most of the extra moves when in the company of his wife. He opens the door for her. He bends to pick up an object that she has dropped. He carries out the trash and mows the lawn.

It's not a bad rule, but under certain circumstances it grants the husband too great an advantage. He gets all the good moves. There are times when he would better demonstrate his love by allowing his wife to get into the action.

In a time of weight equalization, a couple might agree that the one trying to lose weight would make most of the "manner moves." This would mean that sometimes the wife would reach for the fallen object, rise to answer the telephone, or even carry out the trash.

Children can also be blessings that bring back that youthful look. Walking the floor with a crying baby can use up the energy stored at a large evening meal. The weightier mate should always be the one to rise at baby's call. Pushing the stroller around the block will do more to keep a marriage in shape than the daily soap operas.

Running across a field to get a kite airborne is

great exercise. A game of football or shooting a few baskets helps both boys and bulges. Dads who are not very active during the day will need to pace themselves in this. Family fun such as swimming, hiking, or biking has already been suggested, but deserves another mention in this setting.

Ask the Lord for a new attitude toward the experiences in your day that make you go out of your way. The Apostle Paul said thankfulness ought to be a normal reaction. "In everything give thanks; for this is the will of God in Christ Jesus concerning you" (1 Thes. 5:18). Your cheerfulness will give a new atmosphere to your home. You'll end the day with a heart of praise, and will be a healthier person in both mind and body.

The most pleasant avenue open to married losers is simply a revival in their love life. What a delightful way to lose weight!

The couple who sat before me were not young lovers. They were approaching sixty, but had the same stars in their eyes I have seen so many times in those just leaving their teens. They were in love and we were planning their wedding. I turned to the groom and asked where they were going on their honeymoon. "It's going to be a long one," he said. He had the right idea. The one I have been trying to get across to prospective brides and grooms for twenty years.

Why should newlyweds be the greatest lovers? Why shouldn't loving improve with age? Maturity should magnify affection.

The Demonstration of Love
Jesus' lament about the church at Ephesus would be a fitting statement about too many husbands

and wives: "Nevertheless, I have somewhat against thee, because thou has left thy first love" (Rev. 2:4).

Christian couples should remember that their love for each other is to be a demonstration of Christ's love for the church. Your walk of love together should illustrate the love that God has for all men and women. Paul pointed this out to the Ephesian Christians.

> Husbands, love your wives, even as Christ also loved the church, and gave Himself for it, that He might sanctify and cleanse it with the washing of water by the Word; that He might present it to Himself a glorious church, not having spot, or wrinkle, or any such thing; but that it should be holy and without blemish. So ought men to love their wives as their own bodies. He that loveth his wife loveth himself. For no man ever yet hated his own flesh, but nourisheth and cherisheth it, even as the Lord the church; for we are members of His body, of His flesh, and of His bones. For this cause shall a man leave his father and mother, and shall be joined unto his wife, and they two shall be one flesh. This is a great mystery, but I speak concerning Christ and the church. Nevertheless, let every one of you in particular so love his wife even as himself; and the wife see that she reverence her husband (Eph. 5:25-33).

There are, then, some parallels between the love of Christ for the church and the love of a man for his wife that contain valuable lessons for married people.

The love of Christ is a sacrificial love.

A lady once told me that her marriage was completely changed by a preacher's statement He had said, "You may be asking whether or not you are getting enough out of your marriage, when that is not even the question. You should be asking whether or not your husband or wife is getting all that *he* or *she* should be getting out of your marriage." The preacher's thought-provoker had turned their marriage around and had made them givers instead of receivers. And that's what love is all about.

The husband and wife who start looking for ways to please each other will not be disappointed. The whole mood of life will change. And in shaping up their relationship, the accelerated pace will help consume their savings account of unneeded calories.

The love of Christ is an enduring love.

It is sad to meet couples whose love suffered a blow from which it has never recovered. One or the other became offended at some careless word or act and the wound has never healed. Communication died. They are still husband and wife, but only in the legal sense of the word. They smile and seem happy enough in public. Most of their friends do not know about their problem. But when they are alone the wall between them is real.

He comes home at the end of his work day and hides behind the daily paper. He ventures forth long enough to eat his dinner and then retreats to an easy chair to watch television long into the night. They speak occasionally, yet they say little. There is a private nightly marathon to see who can stay up the longest. Finally they retire, exhausted. Another day is over. They have existed.

These two who once stood before a minister to pledge their love now have little in common—

except their size. That has increased with the deepening depression. They have had little to occupy their evenings together aside from junk food and poor entertainment.

How unlike the love of Christ their love has become! He forgives, and forgives again. He is constantly repairing the communication lines as we confess our sins to Him. His love has endured our many failures.

The love of Christ is a love that is expressed often. How long has it been since you expressed your love to your marriage partner? A day? A week? A month? A year? If it has been a long time since you have communicated your love in either word or act, you are not living as God intended.

Keep your love flowing. Look for opportunities to show your love.

What do you like about your wife? Does she cook well? Is she a good housekeeper? Has she given you children? Is she beautiful? Pretty? These and a score of other qualities are excellent excuses to walk across the room and take her in your arms. Every positive point she possesses provides another reason for making love to her.

What is there about your husband that made you choose him to be your man? Is he strong? Gentle? Faithful? Honest? Hardworking? Make a list of his strengths and tell him how much you appreciate them as you give yourself to him tonight.

Does he have weaknesses that irritate you? Don't major on them. Many people have destroyed their marriages by picking away at negatives. Cultivate a positive attitude. You'll find that you reap what you sow. Love communicated will come back to you. Wise Solomon said, "Every wise woman buildeth her house, but the foolish plucketh it down with her hands" (Prov. 14:1).

Do not allow daily distractions to keep you from expressing your love. Pleasing your partner should have priority over petty problems. Paul counseled the Corinthians about this. "Let the husband render unto the wife her due; and likewise also, the wife unto the husband. The wife hath not power of her own body, but the husband; and likewise also the husband hath not power of his own body, but the wife. Defraud ye not one the other, except it be with consent for a time, that Satan tempt you not for your incontinency" (1 Cor. 7:3-5).

Speaking on this portion of Scripture, Dr. Oswald J. Smith explained:

> Your body, God says, is not your own. You thought it was. You withheld it when you should have given it. Husband and wife are one. That body of yours belongs to your husband and his to you, so both have privileges that neither has any right to deny. Have you learned to yield? If there is love, you will.
>
> You say you are too busy, too weary, and too old. Too busy for love? Too weary to express your affection? Too old to yield yourself to the one who loves to hold you in his arms and enjoy your response? Too cold to appreciate the touch of a lover's hand and to express a little of the affection of your heart? Surely not! [1]

What searching questions! How will you answer them?

Perhaps you are not affectionate because your extra weight makes you feel you are not as loveable

---

[1] Oswald J. Smith quoted in *How to Win Your Family for Christ* by Nathaniel Olson, Good News Publishers, 1961, p. 10.

as you once were. That is self-defeating. Frustration, depression, and a push down the road to obesity are the results of that kind of thinking.

Let your love come alive. That is an important part of the abundant life that God intends for you. Both the action and the attitude stimulated by an exciting husband and wife love relationship will help you in all other areas of life. Especially moving will be the incentive to be what your lover wants you to be. And that powerful drive may add just the needed touch to enable you to reach that weight and form you have desired so long.

A calorie
saved
is a
calorie burned.

11 | Share Your Slimming Successes

Now that you're losing weight, tell someone about it.

Voicing your victories will help you win more of them. Share the good news of even the slightest progress. Don't feel that you must wait until you have lost a noticeable amount of weight before telling others. When that time comes, others will be telling you about it. The loss of even a few pounds proves that fat does fall off that frame. You weren't too sure of that. Remember?

Many of God's blessings have started with some small sign. Ignoring or despising that first indication of God's work might have meant the forfeiting of greater things. A good example is the answer to Elijah's prayer for rain after three and one half years of drought. The Bible says that the prophet prayed earnestly, and then sent his servant to see if the clouds were rolling in from the sea. The servant returned saying that he had seen nothing. Finally, after being sent to scan the sky seven more times, he reported, "Behold, there ariseth a little cloud out of the sea, like a man's hand" (1 Kings 18:44).

That encouraging word was enough for Elijah. He ordered that a message be sent to the king telling him that rain was on the way. His weather prediction proved correct. "The heaven was black with clouds and wind, and there was a great rain" (18:45).

So give thanks to God for the loss of that first pound, and find a friend who will be pleased to hear about it. Even if your losses were held to one pound each week, you would be 52 pounds thinner in one year. That's a gain worth getting.

Group Dynamics

The experience of sharing will be made especially easy and helpful in a group situation. There you will be meeting on common ground with others who have a problem similar to yours. The discussion and discovery of mutual struggles will give opportunity to bear one another's burdens. Compassion will grow. You will be pleased when others in the group are successful in losing weight, and your own goal will seem more attainable.

If your church does not have a weight loss class, perhaps you can organize one in the neighborhood. You'll be doing your friends a favor by encouraging them to join.

When we offered this study for the first time in our church, one class member exclaimed, "Thank you for caring!" That expression of appreciation made all the effort of preparation and teaching worthwhile.

The teacher of a weight-loss class can use a

variety of ideas to make the class interesting.

A weekly "weigh-in" keeps everyone alert. The success or failure shared in this ritual can be either hilarious or heartbreaking, depending on diligence in dieting. There is no responsibility without accountability, and facing those scales provides a great incentive to stick with a working program.

Sharing food substitutions can be profitable. It won't take long for a number of losers to be experts on the calorie count of many different dishes. A calorie saved is a calorie burned, so time spent in learning from one another will not be wasted.

Dedicated fat fighters will surprise you in their ingenuity at devising new schemes for adding exercise to the day's routine. Listen to them. Here's an area where many teachers should use that reservoir of inventiveness available in the group.

Sometimes our classes have added up the losses of all the members for a week. This can produce an impressive figure. It's exciting to discover that you have one hundred pounds less fat in the fellowship than you did the previous week. Yet, that is a very reachable goal in a good-sized class.

Be Pleased with Victory

Whether you are in a group or have decided to lose weight as an individual, give thanks to God when telling of your progress. Don't forget that He has made the difference. Think of all those times you tried and failed. Feel again that awful struggle for *will power*. Pinpoint your special areas of victory through Christ and tell your friends about the success He has brought to your pounds-off program. Follow the example of the man whom Jesus healed in Gadara: "And he went his way, and published throughout the whole city what great things Jesus had done unto him (Luke 8:39).

Nancy McKay was in our first weight-loss class. The material we were using at that time was just a skeleton outline of a few pages. Nevertheless, the fundamentals of weight control through a Bible lifestyle were being taught, and she applied them. Consequently, she soon reached her desired weight. She wore clothes that she had not been able to get into for a long time. Her life improved in many ways. She felt more confident. She has since taught some of our Lose Weight the Bible Way classes.

Being publicly pleased with your losses will impress those moments of victory upon your mind. They will be the high points on the road to right weight. And you will need them, for there are persistent, discouraging plateaus along the way. There will be weeks that you will not lose a pound, even though you have done everything right. When those times come you will feel like giving up. Recalling those mountaintops you have shared with others will bolster the optimism and courage you need to carry on.

Talking about your blessings cultivates an attitude of thanksgiving, a frame of mind that keeps success within your reach. It's also spiritually healthy: "It is a good thing to give thanks unto the Lord, and to sing praises unto Thy name, O Most High; to show forth Thy loving-kindness in the morning, and Thy faithfulness every night" (Ps. 92:1-2).

Finally, the thought of losing weight through a Bible formula is foreign to most people. To many, a Bible life-style is visualized as stuffy and stiff.

When you announce that your new look has come out of the old Book, expect a variety of reactions. Be prepared to explain yourself.

Your explanation may be the vehicle that God will use to bring new life to your friends. Most people have no concept of a God who cares about every detail of our lives. To them, He is just Someone up there somewhere. They cannot imagine the Ruler of the universe taking a personal interest in the lives of those who walk on this speck in space called Earth. Even the psalmist wrestled with the reason for it. "When I consider Thy heavens, the work of Thy fingers, the moon and the stars, which Thou hast ordained, what is man, that Thou art mindful of him? And the son of man, that Thou visitest him?" (Ps. 8:3-4)

Yes, God does care. And you know Him personally through His Son, Jesus Christ. You have learned that His love envelopes every part of you: body, soul, and spirit. You are His child, and have the right to call upon Him in all of life's struggles. Now you have discovered that His mighty resources are available to set you free from the tyranny of your own body.

Share that truth.

Your world is waiting to hear it.

It's as easy
as pie
to be back
in the fat fellowship
before you know it.

12

Keep It Off
by
Keeping It Up

Many diet and exercise plans will take off weight. Only a change in life-style will keep it off.

Let's review the reasons for your success in losing weight, whether you have been working at it for several months or are just beginning your adventure.

You now understand your responsibility to keep your body at its best. It is the temple of God. You have a new respect for your earthly house. You know that God cares about your appearance and health, as well as your soul.

You have discovered that the key to successful dieting is the dieter. You are now a calorie counter and have become adept at allowing yourself variety and nutrition without exceeding the feed limit.

You have learned to watch for the first signs of depression. You have been avoiding situations that trigger despair. You know that depression is a diet destroyer and, consequently, you have kept your thought patterns positive as much as possible.

Satan has been unmasked. You're aware of his purpose to ruin your health and effectiveness, and you're alert to his approaches when food is around.

Faith has made a difference in your figure. Had it not been for the confidence that with God all things are possible, you might still be carrying that load of extra weight that you neither needed nor wanted.

Self-control. How good it was to find that you could have it through the power of the Holy Spirit. Your will power has been weighed and found wanting during so many weight loss attempts in the past.

And exercise. You never knew there were so many opportunities for it. New ones appear every day, now that you're looking for them.

Living intensely has made it possible to accomplish so much more. You've been plunging into life and enjoying it.

You're active and involved in Christian service. It isn't necessary to coax you to use your gifts and abilities anymore. You feel challenged in life.

Your home is different because you have become a giver instead of a receiver. Love lives at your house again.

Your friends are pleased with your new attitude and appearance. You're telling others about God's blessings in this very personal area of your life and it's opening doors to share the message of Christ with them.

The Old Life-style

Sometimes you wonder what happened to that discouraged, overweight individual who some time ago started out to lose weight the Bible way.

If you miss him, let me tell you 11 ways to bring him back.

1. Stop caring about your body.
2. Eat all you want of whatever you crave. Often.
3. Feel sorry for yourself and try to capture the pity of your friends and family. Enjoy being down.
4. Conclude that the devil doesn't exist, or that he only operates in taverns and dance halls.
5. Stop praying and trusting God about the needs and condition of your body. Get too spiritual for that.
6. If you ever get the urge to lose a few pounds, do it on your own. You've got a lot of will power. You can do it.
7. Sleep an extra hour each morning and catch a nap every afternoon. Cut out those calisthenics. A busy person like you can't spare the time. Save steps whenever you can. Make the children run all the errands. You're not getting any younger, you know.
8. Ease up on your enthusiasm. Who'll know the difference in a thousand years? Trying to impress somebody? Don't you know you'll raise the standard on your job? Relax.
9. Resign from your Sunday School class. Quit the choir. Let the pastor do the visiting in the community. That's what he's paid to do. Don't make any promises about work around the church. You might not be able to keep them and then you'll be a liar. You know what the Bible says about liars.
10. Start demanding your rights at home. You've been doing all the giving long enough. It's

about time things started coming your way
for a change. Pout till she produces. Clam
up. She'll come around.

11. Despise discipline. It's a free country. Live
as you please. All you get out of life is what
you eat, so make the best of it.

That's all. It's as easy as pie. You'll be back in
the fat fellowship before you know it. All those
clothes that you put away when the fat started falling off will have to be pressed into service again.
And you'll be longing to lose, just like old times.

Frightening? I should think so. Yet, it is all too
true.

Your New Life-style

Thankfully, you don't have to return to your portly
past. The same life-style that brought you to your
desired weight will keep you there: The disciplined
Christian lifestyle.

"That sounds like I'll have to live with self-
discipline all my life," you say.

That's right. Listen to the testimony of another
disciplined Christian: "But I keep under my body,
and bring it into subjection" (1 Cor. 9:27).

"Sounds like a life of self-denial," you groan.

Right again. And doesn't that have a familiar
ring? "And when He had called the people unto
Him with His disciples also, He said unto them,
'Whosoever will come after Me, let him deny him-
self, and take up his cross, and follow Me'"
(Mark 8:34).

So, it's true. A Bible life-style is disciplined and
different. Not unpleasant, but different. Some reject it. Nevertheless, it has produced wonderful results in your life. And isn't it nice to walk by a

mirror and experience that feeling of accomplishment. You and Jesus have achieved something.

Of course you'll want to adjust your new life-style slightly when you arrive at your goal. You can't go on losing weight too long. So to level off you will have to experiment a bit. If your weight continues to drop you should eat more than you did while you were trying to lose. It may also be necessary to trim a small amount of action from your daily routine.

Keep an eye on those scales for now. In a matter of weeks you'll know your limit. After that, constant weight watching won't be quite so important, providing you stick with your new way of life. Even so, a weekly weighing will be wise. Body changes may require more fine tuning, and any abrupt loss or gain without change in your food intake or in your activity should send you to your doctor.

I have purposely used the word *life-style* a number of times in this chapter. When you have succeeded in losing your excess weight, I suggest that you drop the word *diet* from your vocabulary. You are no longer trying to recover from obesity, or an overweight condition. You are now well, and intend to live in a manner that will keep you from being afflicted in that way again. You have adopted a new life-style.

Expect public reaction.

Before, when you turned down chocolate cake, blueberry pie, or some other delicious dessert, most of your friends understood. Many may have admired your effort. Now it will be different. Some hostesses, beholding your trim shape, may conclude that you are not eating their offerings because you are not satisfied with the food. Consistency is the only remedy for that reaction. When it becomes clear that you *always* refuse desserts and other calorie-rich foods, the cooks will not be offended.

Finally, keep your motives right.

Losing weight and keeping it off to attract attention and draw people to yourself is wrong. Even so, the possibility of this pitfall should never be an excuse for obesity. You can keep your reasons for reducing right.

Weigh your motives in a prayerful manner. Ask the Lord for a proper attitude. Keep your heart right with a daily conditioning in the Bible. There are many portions of Scripture that deal with the pride problem. Solomon said a lot about it. "The fear of the Lord is to hate evil; pride, and arrogance, and the evil way, and the perverse mouth, do I hate" (Prov. 8:13). "When pride cometh, then cometh shame; but with the lowly is wisdom" (11:2). "Pride goeth before destruction, and an haughty spirit before a fall" (16:18). "A man's pride shall bring him low, but honor shall uphold the humble in spirit" (29:23).

Don't let pride be your motivation for losing weight. Instead, let His praise be the purpose of your project. His glory the reason for your new life-style: "Whether, therefore, ye eat, or drink, or whatever ye do, do all to the glory of God" (1 Cor. 10:31).